The 2027 Chiropractic Textbook

Volume 3

Claude Lessard, D.C.

www.LessardChiropractic.com
Lessard Chiropractic Center
210 Makefield Road, Morrisville, PA 19067
215-736-8816

DEDICATION

JOSEPH B. STRAUSS, D.C., F.C.S.C.

There is no doubt that the singular blessing of Joseph in my life is the fruit of his true and tireless capacity to know and facilitate a greater understanding of the chiropractic philosophy. Innumerable and extended conversations refined several key ideas in "The 2027 Chiropractic Textbook," especially this present Volume 3. Almost 50 years of deep and dedicated exchanges between us have served to elucidate the foundation the chiropractic philosophy as given us by D.D. and B.J. Palmer, showing it to be both "ancient" and "ever new." Countless hours about the innate law of living things being the point of praxis – where chiropractic philosophy truly begins in practice – proved the catalyst in defining the vertebral subluxation as the specific interference in the momentum of TRANSMISSION of innate impulses for coordination of activities.

Our collective vision always admitted of the research and information contained in the Blue Books as an irreplaceable tool of the teaching compendium of every chiropractic institution. The thrust of his focus and insight gave evidence of his brilliant intellect. His goal in constructing an ever-clearer working knowledge of the philosophy was to form and fuel future generations of chiropractic minds. What drove such personal self-sacrifice was the conviction that chiropractic thinking informed by this new information would translate into an ever deeper understanding of the chiropractic objective. The premise of all the ideas we explored was the shared conviction that our profession stands at a crossroad.

Every chiropractor, without condemnation, has the stunning and unique opportunity to move from the outright and deeply personal values of our founders to the elemental foundation of chiropractic itself: to embrace its universal values, the 33 principles of chiropractic basic science!

In dedicating Volume 3 of "The 2027 Chiropractic Textbook" to Joseph B. Strauss, D.C., F.C.S.C., I acknowledge with gratitude his unparalleled contribution to me personally and to our beloved profession.

We share the hope that fortified by the vision espoused in his living legacy, the Blue Books will continue guiding the profession, present and future, to choose to practice exclusively the pure, unadulterated chiropractic objective.

TABLE OF CONTENTS

PREFACE

This is a series of four academic volumes to be studied as part of the chiropractic curriculum for the student to learn chiropractic and graduate as a chiropractor. It is the 2027 reconstructed version of its original precursor, "CHIROPRACTIC TEXT BOOK" written by Ralph W. Stephenson, D.C. in 1927. This is the third volume of the series, what Stephenson calls the "Junior Text." Portions of this volume are taken directly from the original text and updated with NEW knowledge produced from NEW information of the last hundred years. The same building blocks of chiropractic are deconstructed, reorganized, and reconstructed into a contemporary context that includes 130 years of continuous discoveries. Credit is given to D.D. Palmer, D.C., B.J. Palmer, D.C., and R.W. Stephenson, D.C.. We all stand on their shoulders as we move forward.

I applied to Sherman College in December of 1973. I was first introduced to the founder of Sherman College, Thom Gelardi, D.C. during the orientation day. Over the years, Thom and I developed a close relationship. After hundreds of hours of conversation, it was at his suggestion, in the early summer of 2021 that I undertook the task of rewriting the chiropractic textbook.

I owe much to Reggie Gold, D.C. for facilitating the formation of my chiropractic mind and for always encouraging me to THINK and THINK and THINK. I am grateful to Reggie for his constant challenges that stretched me to this day to grasp the unadulterated aspect of the exclusivity of the chiropractic objective.

I have no doubt that without the constant affirmation, encouragement, and deep friendship of Joseph Strauss, D.C., The 2027 Chiropractic Textbook could never have been rewritten.

My heartfelt gratitude goes James Healey, D.C. for continuously being my devil's advocate, asking the questions that provide a needed accuracy check to my philosophical contemplation. His constant desire for authentic articulation to facilitate understanding is a true inspiration. Thank you, Jim.

Thank you to Tom Gregory, D.C. for your steady listening and comments on the philosophical exactitude of the text.

Thank you to Jack Bourla, D.C. for the specific chiropractic editing of Volume 2 and 3 into a comprehensive academic text. Your questions, contributions, and insightful scribblings in the margins of the drafts, fueled thoughts that have instigated clearer description of difficult material.

Thank you to Judy Campenale, D.C. for providing me with my weekly spinal checks. I am eternally grateful to you for so many long hours of meaningful conversation about new insights that were instrumental in writing Volumes 1, 2 and 3.

I owe an immense gratitude to Amanda Janiec, my Executive Assistant, for overseeing the entire project and making it possible. As Amanda tackled the English editing of the manuscripts with judicious research for the proper references in the text, making sure I was accurate, she became my radar following the text through her scholarly perspective. She is truly a most trusted executive assistant. Thank you Amanda for your dedication and for sharing your educated expertise.

Finally, to the one and only person who saw me through it all, Sara, my spouse of fifty years, without whom I could not be the person that I am today. From the very beginning of translating my phonetic notes of our first quarter at Sherman, she never wavered and has always been true. I love you, Sara.

These volumes are mainly "The Chiropractic Text Book" originally written by R.W. Shephenson, D.C. They include error corrections and are updated with NEW knowledge of the past hundred years. The instructions contained therein are further developed from the original concepts of the founder of chiropractic, Daniel David Palmer, D.C. and his son, the developer of chiropractic, Bartlett Joshua Palmer, D.C.. Within these volumes, the falsification and deconstruction of the theistic and anthropomorphic characters given to some of the chiropractic's scientific principles and scientific laws, namely universal intelligence and innate intelligence, are proven. Those chiropractic concepts are then reconstructed on the solid bedrock of the testable and verifiable principles of chiropractic's basic science; they include new information acquired since 1927 that dictates the chiropractic objective. These four volumes contain NEW knowledge that has been discovered and constructed, within the past 100 years, from NEW information that was unavailable from 1895 to 1927 and beyond. They cover the philosophy, the science, and the art of chiropractic. They are intended to be a further study of chiropractic that is continuously developed to CARRY ON the genius of our predecessors, D.D. and B.J. Palmer into the 21st century. They are designed to convey more precisely "WHAT" chiropractic is, "HOW" to apply its scientific principles, and the hard to vary explanation of "WHY" chiropractic is an evolutionary humanitarian approach to EVERY experience of life, not just the experience of health. These volumes comprise error corrections that are necessary for the student to obtain an assured confidence in the chiropractic objective including its universal value. They honor yet modernize this significant discovery and the greater understanding of its necessary and humanitarian service to the world. It was Joseph B. Strauss, D.C. who wrote in 2002, "I do not believe that you can truly understand chiropractic philosophy without studying Stephenson. There are truths within and errors that need to be seen and understood for any student to ever begin to reach a level of comprehension of chiropractic as it was and is today."[1] Students are encouraged to study Stephenson's textbook of 1927, ALL of the Strauss' Blue Books, and the Blue Books that I have personally authored, *A New Look at Chiropractic's Basic Science , Timed Out: Chiropractic, and The 2027 Chiropractic Textbook Volume 1 and 2.*

It is the hope that the truths and error corrections contained within the pages of these volumes will inform and inspire future generations of chiropractors so that they can make an informed choice in constructing their professional mission. Based on the study of the 33 principles of chiropractic's basic science, it is crystal clear that the sole aim of the chiropractic objective is, EXCLUSIVELY: the restoration of the transmission of innate impulses through the location, analysis, and the facilitation of the correction of vertebral subluxations. PERIOD.

These texts have been written for educational instruction. They are divided into Volume One (First Year Chiropractic Text), Volume Two (Second Year Chiropractic Text), Volume Three (Third Year Chiropractic Text), and Volume Four (Fourth Year Chiropractic Text). Following the original layout of Stephenson's Text Book allows for the integral comparison of topics. There are questions for review that are intended to help the student THINK and REFLECT in order to "internalize" the universal value of chiropractic, and raise inquiry to test any of its 33 scientific principles for validation or falsification. The student is urged to become familiar with the unique chiropractic lexicon at the beginning of every volume in order to properly understand the meaning of those terms that will undoubtedly assist the study of the text. Hopefully, these four volumes of the updated chiropractic textbook will encourage future chiropractors to CARRY ON and further develop chiropractic, that will include NEW knowledge, insights, and error corrections into the third millennium and forever more.

---

1. Strauss, Joseph. "The Green Book Commentaries, Vol. XIV (1927) Chiropractic Text Book." Levittown, PA: Foundation for Advancement of Chiropractic Education. (2002). p.17

CHIROPRACTIC LEXICON

GLOSSARY

In order to continue to explore the previously established central core of chiropractic, namely its principles and tenets, in a contemporary way we must rely on a base set terminology. As we move forward our educated intelligence grows and it requires that we progress without condemnation. The following glossary of terms was compiled, with the help of Joseph B. Strauss, D.C., many of which are originally from Stephenson's text. Some additional terms that are uniquely needed for practicing the chiropractic objective have been incorporated.

100%/perfect: A quality of being free from all flaws or defect. It is the fullness of something material or immaterial.

Adaptability (sign of life): The intrinsic ability that a living organism possesses to act on all information/force, which comes to it whether innate or universal.

Adaptation: The movement of a living organism or any of its parts, or the structural change in that organism, to use or to circumvent environmental information/force. Adaptation is a continuous process — continually varying, it is never constant and unvarying, as are other universal laws. Adaptation is a universal principle — the only one of its kind. It is the principle of change and the change is always according to law, which is 100%/perfect instantaneous integral adaptation.

ADIO (Acronym for Above-Down-Inside-Out):

1. An exclusive model of world viewpoint, under which chiropractic philosophy, logically and uncompromisingly, exists.

2. A thinking process with a unique perspective on life. First, there are absolutes in life (Prin. 1, 6, 20). Second, everything has a cause that should be addressed, if possible (Prin. 17, 24). Third, there is a pre-eminence to the educated intelligence of humankind (Prin. 22, 27), a 100%/perfect universal intelligence (Prin. 1,5).

3. Life comes from universal organization ABOVE (Prin. 1, 3), DOWN to living things' innate adaptation (Prin. 20, 23), expressing signs of life INSIDE the body (Prin. 18), to be manifested OUT as a living entity (Prin. 21).

4. In regards to coordination of activities of body parts (Prin. 32), in the vertebrate body, the innate impulse flows from the brain cell ABOVE (Prin. 28), DOWN to the tissue cell below (Prin. 18), is expressed from INSIDE the body part (Prin. 21), to be manifested OUT as coordinative purpose (Prin. 21, 32), according to universal laws (Prin. 24).

ADIO analysis: A specific method of chiropractic analysis based on the principles of chiropractic's basic science i.e., that the function of the innate law is always normal (Prin. 27); that the innate law will adapt and organize para-vertebral muscles to process a vertebral adjustment, thus correcting a vertebral subluxation to restore to innate-normal the transmission of innate impulses for coordination of activities within the limitation of E/matter (Prin. 23, 24, 31a, 31b). The chiropractor's pre-check is to objectively measure indicators of a vertebral subluxation, and to palpate in order to identify the vectors of the correcting muscles of a vertebral subluxation processed through the innate law, which reveal when and where a vertebral subluxation exists. This pre-check is performed for the appropriate introduction of a specific adjustic thrust to facilitate the processing of a vertebral adjustment by the innate law. The chiropractor's post-check is to recheck the objective indicators of the vertebral subluxation and to palpate those same muscles to determine if the vertebral subluxation has been corrected.

Adjustic thrust: An adjustic thrust is a specific, external, educated information/force introduced at the site of a subluxated vertebra with the intent that the innate law of living things will process a vertebral adjustment to correct a vertebral subluxation.

Afferent nerve: The nerve that transmits trophic impulses/signals from receptor tissue cell to central processing brain cell for coordination of activities. It is the route of feedback information/force from tissue cell to brain cell. It is not to be confused with sensory nerves, which transmit sensory impulses from sense organs to physical brain.

Analytical post-check: The end-point of a chiropractic analysis to determine if the correction of a vertebral subluxation has occurred. It is the completion of practicing the chiropractic objective.

Analytical pre-check: The start-point of a chiropractic analysis that locates and identifies the vectors of the corrective muscles working to correct a vertebral subluxation in order to introduce to it a specific adjustic thrust to facilitate its correction by the innate law.

Angular momentum: The total fluctuating motion of intra-cell particulates of the neuron-transmitters. It can be interfered by vertebral subluxations, thus altering the transmission of the innate impulse.

Assimilation (a sign of life): The ability of a living organism, through the innate law, to selectively take food materials into its body and make them a part of itself according to a systematic program designed by a universal intelligence (Prin. 18).

Characterization: The construction of specific codes by the universal principle of organization that organizes universal information/force in order to maintain energy/matter in existence; it is also the reconstruction (modified for living energy/matter) of specific codes by the innate law of living things that adapts universal information/force into innate information/force.

Chiropractic analysis: A chiropractic analysis is the act of examining the nerve system and the vertebral column in detail, to locate and identify the vectors of the corrective muscles working to correct a vertebral subluxation, in order to introduce a specific adjustic thrust to facilitate the processing of a vertebral adjustment by the innate law.

Chiropractic Meaning of Existence: It is the expression of the universal principle of organization through all energy/matter (Prin. 2).

Chiropractic objective: The chiropractic objective is to locate, analyze, and facilitate the correction of vertebral subluxations for an innate-normal transmission of the innate impulses of the body. PERIOD. The chiropractic objective is derived directly from the thirty-three principles of chiropractic's basic science. Nothing more. Nothing less. Nothing else.

Chiropractor: "One who knows the science, art and philosophy of Chiropractic and how to adjust subluxated vertebrae by placing in apposition the articular processes of the vertebral column."[2]

Chiropractor's vision: The chiropractor's vision is to ensure the availability of chiropractic care to EVERYONE throughout their lifetime.

---

2. Palmer, B.J., " The Science of Chiropractic, Its Principles and Philosophies." 4th ed., Davenport, IA: The Palmer School of Chiropractic-Chiropractic Fountain Head. (1920) p. 12

Coding: The assignment of specific characters to identify a specific communication system programmed to construct a message.

Computation: The operation of a computing system. It is the processing of data of a computing system using a software program.

Copyability: The ability to be copied, to be duplicatable. From the maxim that "One cannot give what one does not have." Every human invention is a copy of something already existing in principle. The universe is complete.

Counterfactuals: They are facts not about what is "actual" but about what is possible or not possible. For example, Dead Sea scrolls exist somewhere "hidden" on our planet. That is a physical property of those scrolls since they do exist. That it ***could be possible*** to read the words on them is a counterfactual property regardless of whether those scrolls would ever be discovered. And yet that those words *could be* read would still be true.

De-coding: To convert a coded message into intelligible language that can be understood.

Disease and DIS-EASE: Disease is a term used by physicians for sickness. To them it is an entity and is worthy of a name, hence diagnosis. DIS-EASE is a chiropractic term meaning not having ease; or lack of ease. It is lack of an entity. It is a condition of energy/matter when it does not have the property of ease. Ease is the entity, and DIS-EASE the lack of it.

E/matter: This term means energy-matter. Since $E=mc^2$, energy and matter are equivalent and interchangeable; energy is simply a different configuration (properties) of electrons, protons, and neutrons with varying velocities (activities). For example, water has 2 atoms of hydrogen and 1 atom of oxygen, whether it is in a fluid state, ice state, or vapor/gas state. It is dependent upon the motion of its basic elements. It is a term reminding us that energy and matter are equivalent and interchangeable as per $E=mc^2$, and that matter is comprised of electrons, protons, and neutrons configured at less than the square of the speed of light.

Educated brain/field: That part of the brain used by innate law of living things, as an organ, for reason, will, memory, education, and the voluntary functions.

Educated control: Educated control (also known as educated mind) is the activity of innate law of living things in the educated brain as an organ. The output of this activity is educated impulses such as thoughts, reasoning, will, memory, etc... The innate law of living things controls the functions of the voluntary systems via the educated brain. Educated impulses are modified innate impulses (tinctured) that have passed through the educated brain and are mostly for adaptation to things external to the body.

Educated impulse: The innate information/force through the educated brain that becomes modified with whatever quality the educated mind can give it for the voluntary functions of the body. Note that the educated brain "controls" nothing, except that the innate information/force passes through it. Adaptation of information/force is ALWAYS and ONLY through the coding of innate information/force by the innate law. When innate impulses pass through the educated brain, they are "tinctured" so as to be modified into educated impulses for conscious action.

Educated Intelligence: The capability of the educated brain to function. It starts at 0% at birth and reaches its maximum limit at the death of the body (since it will develop no further).

Educated information/force: Educated information/force is innate information/force that has been modified by the educated mind for voluntary functions. It is really an educated impulse.

Efferent nerve: The transmitting nerve of innate impulses from the central processing brain cell to the receptor tissue cell. It is the route of conducted innate information/force from brain cell to tissue cell.

Energy: Electrons, protons, and neutrons configured at the square of the speed of light ($E=mc^2$).

E/matter: Energy/matter is electrons, protons, and neutrons configured at specific velocities in time.

Existence: The continuous motion of elemental particles of E/matter (Prin. 14).

External educated information/force: An external educated information/force is innate information/force that has been voluntarily modified by the educated intelligence with a new educated character for voluntary action with a definite purpose. Ex: An adjustic thrust.

Factorial moment: A factorial moment is a moment generating function computed by the innate law of living things for adaptive organization of the body of a living thing through instantaneous integral adaptation within the limitation of E/matter and time.

Flow: The action of something moving along in a steady continuous stream. In the body, it is the smooth continuous movement of information/F from one place to another.

Growth (a sign of life): Growth is the ability of a living organism to expand according to intelligent programming to mature in size and is dependent upon the power of assimilation (Prin. 18).

Hard to vary explanation: An explanation that provides specific details that fit together so tightly that it is impossible to change any detail without affecting its whole. In the case of chiropractic, the principles of its basic science are the hard to vary explanation of chiropractic.

Impression: The information/force coded by the innate law as trophic impulses/signals, based on the complexity of the tissue cell concerning its soundness and functions.

Information/F: Information/force are computed and coded instructions to configure electrons, protons, neutrons, and their velocities. Information/force is organized by the principle of organization (Prin. 8).

Inforuns: Inforuns, (also known as foruns) are non-discrete information/force units that are continually organized by the universal principle of organization providing properties and actions to all E/matter in order to *maintain* it in existence (Prin. 1, 8). Inforuns must be adapted by the innate law of living things and to be reconstructed into innate impulses for coordination of activities of all the parts of the body, or into innate rays/waves for cellular metabolism in order to *maintain* E/matter alive (Prin. 21, 23).

Innate control: Innate control (also known as innate mind) is the activity of the innate law in the innate field. It is the introduction of innate instructive information/F, as governance, into E/matter via the innate field of the body of *living* things to *maintain* the material of the body alive if it is possible according to universal laws within the limits of adaptation (Prin. 21, 24).

Innate field: The innate field (also known as innate brain) is:

a) That aspect of the living body used by the innate law of living things, as an operating system, in which to adapt universal information/F and assemble them,

b) That facet of a living organism controlled by the innate law of living things, as an operating system, in which to assemble innate impulses, innate rays or innate waves, trophic impulses, and sensory impulses.

Innate impulse: Innate impulse (also known as mental impulse) is a unit of information/F for a specific body part, for a specific function, for coordination of activities. A specific instruction given to a body part, for coordination of activities, for the present moment.

Innate information/F: Innate information/force (also known as innate force) is universal information/force adapted by the innate law of living things and codified for use in the body. It is assembled for dynamic functional process within the innate field to cause tissue cells to function or to offer resistance to the environment. It is transmitted by nerve conduction from the brain to the tissue cell and is called an *innate impulse* when it impels parts of the body for coordinated action; it is called an *educated impulse* for voluntary actions; it is called a *trophic impulse/signal* for feedback from the state and coordination of activities of body parts to the brain; it is called an *innate ray/wave* when it is radiated from within all cells of the body for metabolism; and it is called a *sensory impulse* when it is transmitted by sensory nerve from the environment, via sense organs, to the brain for adaptation to environmental circumstances for every factorial moments. Innate information/F is constructive toward structural E/matter (Prin. 26). Chiropractic ONLY addresses the transmission of the innate impulse for coordination of activities of body parts. Chiropractic does NOT address the educated impulse, the trophic impulse, the innate ray/wave.

Innate law of living things: The innate law of living (also known as innate intelligence) is the inborn organizing principle that governs the body of a living thing through adaptation in order to *maintain* it alive, only if it is possible according to universal laws. It is the essential extension of the universal principle of organization that is keeping living E/matter alive through multiple levels of complex organization. It implements design, programming, self-correction, adjustability and adaptation to internal and external effectors.

Innate ray/wave: A unit of information/F for a specific tissue cell unit to keep it metabolically sound and alive for a specific unit of time within limitations of E/matter.

Instantaneous integral adaptation: Instantaneous integral adaptation (also known as intellectual adaptation) is the 100%/perfect cooperative processes of the innate law of living things to compute ways and means of adapting universal information/F and E/matter for use in the body and for coordination of activities. The interoperability of the innate law, in the innate field, to keep ALL the complexities of the living things organized to *maintain* it alive if it is possible according to universal laws (Prin. 21, 23, 24).

Instantiation: The act of producing a specific application of a principle. It is a process to deduce an individual statement from a general principle; the representation of an idea in the form of an instance of it.

Interoperability: A characteristic of the innate law in the innate field adapting and computing information/F, the interface of which is completely understood to work with ALL the systems of the body, at present or in the future, every factorial moment in either implementation or access (Prin. 33).

Intra-cell particulates: Components of a cell adapted through innate information/F, in the form of innate rays/waves, that have been specifically coded by the innate law to process innate-normal metabolism (Prin. 27) for soundness of the cell.

Invasive information/F: Universal information/F acting powerfully upon tissue in spite of the internal resistance of the body, or in cases where the resistance of the body is lowered.

Logic: Logic in chiropractic is the integration of concepts into the total sum of knowledge acquired through reflective thinking without contradictory identification.

Matter: Electrons, protons, and neutrons configured at *less* that the square of the speed of light.

Mission of the chiropractic profession: The mission of the chiropractic profession is the specific task of increasing the awareness of the UNIVERSAL values of chiropractic for EVERYONE through education and by EXCLUSIVELY practicing the chiropractic objective.

Modifier: A slight change (tincture) transforming a specific code through educated control that manifests innate impulses into educated impulses for voluntary functions.

Momentum: The possession of motion that is compounded by the mass of E/matter moved and its velocity. It is the active movement of E/matter in time. In chiropractic, momentum is the active frequencies of motion of the transmitting E/matter (neuron-transmitters) within the vertebrate body. Mass x Velocity = Momentum. Also, momentum is subject to interference through being transferred from one element of information/F to another by vertebral subluxations. The *total* momentum of E/matter of the living body is always conserved.

Motor nerve: The nerve that transmits educated impulses (modified innate impulses) from the central processing brain cell to the receptor tissue cell. It is the route of educated functions from brain cell to tissue cell for voluntary actions.

Myo-vector: A chiropractic term describing the directional work of an operating para-vertebral muscle, adapted by the innate law, to process a vertebral adjustment for the correction of a vertebral subluxation within the limitations of E/matter (Prin. 23, 24, 31a, 31b). Utilized in ADIO analysis, a myo-vector reveals that the vertebra is not, at that moment, correctly positioned and is interfering with the transmission of innate impulses.

Objective Chiropractic Movement: The Objective Chiropractic Movement holds that: The practice of the chiropractic objective exists as a complete objective having universal value based on the application of the 33 principles of chiropractic's basic science which is independent of the chiropractor's feelings, wishes, hopes or fears.

Objective chiropractor (OC): An Objective Chiropractor is one who chooses to practice EXCLUSIVELY the chiropractic objective and nothing else.

Penetrative information/F: Invasive information/F that acts powerfully assailing the body and that has effect upon tissue in spite of the internal resistance of the body.

Physical brain: That part of the central nerve system used by the innate law of living things, as an organ, to centralize innate impulses that will be conducted across nerves for distribution to all the parts of the body for coordination of actions (Prin. 28). It is also the organ of adaptation including the faculties of memory, will, and reason.

Poison: Any substance introduced into or manufactured within the living body, which the innate law of living things cannot process for metabolism.

Principle: A fundamental truth that is the foundation of universal laws.

Purpose of chiropractic: The purpose of chiropractic is to restore the momentum of transmission of innate impulses through the location, analysis and facilitation of the correction of vertebral subluxations.

Reflective thinking: Reflective thinking is a process of identification and integration; it is being able to observe oneself from the inside-out, which means to see what's going on inside and outside of oneself.

It is a way to be transparent as regard to one's personal opinionated ideas. It requires not only critical thinking, but being open to flexibility and self-correction by continuously reassessing one's original, personal assumptions. In chiropractic, reflective thinking is an active, persistent, continuous, and careful consideration of the 33 principles of chiropractic's basic science, including its deductive conclusion.

Resistive information/F: Internal innate information/F that opposes invasive or penetrative information/F. It may manifest in many forms, physical, chemical, or mechanical. It is not called resistive information/F unless it is of that character. It is necessary for keeping ALL information/F in balance within the body.

Sensory nerve: The nerve that transmits sensory impulses from the perceptible tissue cell sensor to the brain cell processor. It is the route of special sense functions from the external impressions detected by a tissue cell sensor to a brain cell processor to adapt to the environment, not to be confused with the afferent nerves used for feedback for coordination of activities.

Tone: Tone is the degree of ease manifested by the neurons of the specific nerves that are engaged in he transmission of innate impulses. "Tone is the normal degree of *nerve* tension. Tone is expressed in functions by the normal elasticity, activity, strength and excitability of *nerves* which are too tense or too slack."[25]

Trophic impulse/signal: Information/F that has been characterized and coded by the innate law providing specific feedback information of the metabolic and coordinative state of a tissue cell. A trophic impulse/signal is transmitted through afferent nerves from tissue cell to brain cell via its cell body waving it signal through the innate field for coordination of activities. Not to be confused with the sensory nerves.

Universal information/F: Information/F organized *by* the universal principle of organization that is manifested by physical laws; it provides properties and actions to all E/matter that maintains it in existence (Prin. 1); it is deconstructive toward structural E/matter (Prin. 26).

Universal intelligence: The fundamental CAUSE in chiropractic. Philosophically, it is the capability of the universal principle of organization to organize all of the infinite information/F, in the universal field to provide the properties and the actions of all E/matter *maintaining* it in existence (Prin. 1). It is the cause of organization due to the fact that organization bespeaks intelligence.

Universal principle of organization: The fundamental principle (major premise) of chiropractic's basic science intrinsic to all E/matter. The universal principle of organization is continually organizing all information/F expressed E/matter that supplies all properties and actions to all E/matter in order to maintain it in existence. It is the initial condition of chiropractic's basic science that maintains E/matter in existence (Prin. 1).

Vertebral adjustment and chiropractic adjustment: A vertebral adjustment is the correction of a vertebral subluxation caused by the process of adapting information/F by the innate law of living things Prin. 31a, 31b). A chiropractic adjustment is the application of an adjustic thrust by a chiropractor, at the specific site of a vertebral subluxation, with the intent that the innate law will adapt this specific educated information/F to process a vertebral adjustment.

Viability: The capability of E/matter to live.

---

25. Palmer, D.D., "Text-Book of the Science, Art, and Philosophy of Chiropractic for Students and Practioners." Portland, OR: Portland Printing House Company. (1910) p.7

Vibration: The motion of a tissue cell performing its function.

Vitality: The soundness or integrity of a tissue cell. It is the quality of liveliness of a cell.

CRUCIAL CLARIFICATIONS

Now that you are half way through your course of chiropractic study, you are ready to understand some distinctions between chiropractic's purpose and chiropractic's objective, and between your profession's vision and your profession's mission. It is extremely important to differentiate those four identifications (elemental distinctions) and to integrate them in your repertoire of knowledge.

The Merriam-Webster dictionary defines *purpose* as "the reason for which something is done or for which something exists." The chiropractic purpose is its "raison d'être." It is what chiropractic is, its universal nature, its universal value. It is what chiropractic is intended for. It is the **"WHAT"** of chiropractic. The purpose of chiropractic is to restore the momentum of transmission of innate impulses through the location, analysis, and facilitation of the correction of vertebral subluxations. Chiropractic's purpose is inherent to the principles of its basic science, which is the instructive information guiding chiropractors to apply in order to practice the chiropractic objective. These guiding principles of chiropractic's basic science require no external justification. They have intrinsic universal values, meanings, and relevance to our conduct as professionals. Chiropractic's purpose is the physical manifestation of continuous coordination of activities of the body. Chiropractic is the philosophy, the science and the art of specifically locating, analyzing and correcting vertebral subluxations in accordance with the principles of its basic science (*See Art. 2*).

The Merriam-Webster dictionary defines *objective* as "not influenced by personal feelings or opinions in considering and representing facts; something toward which effort is directed: an end of action." The chiropractic objective is the location, analysis and facilitation of the correction of vertebral subluxations for an innate-normal transmission of the innate impulses of the body. The start-point of chiropractic is its initial condition, its fundamental principle; it is the universal principle of organization. Then, the chiropractic objective is the end-point of chiropractic. The chiropractic objective focuses on a specific cause of interference in transmission of conducted innate information/F for coordination of activities (the vertebral subluxation) and the correction of the interference (Prin. 31a, 31b). Chiropractic is about the innate-normal transmission of innate impulses for coordination of activities of all the parts of the body. The chiropractic objective is not about effects. The chiropractic objective is not influenced by personal values or individual opinions. It is not dependent on the educated control for its existence. The chiropractic objective is universal because the chiropractic objective is derived from the principle of chiropractic's basic science. It is chiropractic philosophy that explain why the chiropractic objective is what it is and does what it does. It is the **"WHY"** of chiropractic. Chiropractors practicing the chiropractic objective may rest assured that they are always staying on track, on course and not deviating, because the chiropractic objective is deduced from the 33 principles of chiropractic's basic science. The 33 principles of chiropractic's basic science are absolute, immutable and constant. As our educated intelligence evolves and our understanding grows, they may be refined. They form the solid bedrock on which the structural nature of chiropractic stands.

The Merriam-Webster dictionary defines *vision* as "the act or power of imagination; the ability to think about the future with wisdom." The chiropractic profession's vision is based on the understanding of "WHAT" will never change, and "HOW" the manner in which chiropractors practice their art should be open to change should new current information become available. The vision is to insure the availability of chiropractic to everyone forever. This vision is authentic and genuine because "WHAT" chiropractic is will never change. It is "WHAT" it is. The vision may be refined, but never change. Chiropractic is the philosophy, the science and the art of specifically locating, analyzing and correcting vertebral subluxations in accordance with the principles of its basic science (*See Art. 2*). It is its very nature, its core ideology, "WHAT" it is. The vision is what we stand for, who we are as a profession and why we exist as professionals. The vision forms who we are as an entity, as a profession. "WHAT" chiropractic is cannot be changed regardless of individual preferences, state laws, countries, culture or personal values. Chiropractic is comprised of universal values. Our professional vision is who we say we are and do what we do. Our vision is the lasting qualities that will remain the same over the course of our lifetime. The vision is what we aspire to achieve as core values and inspires us. The consistency with which we embody our vision is what makes our profession separate and distinct, determining who we are as a profession. The chiropractic profession's vision is to insure the availability of chiropractic care to everyone from this point on.

The Merriam-Webster dictionary defines *mission* as "a specific task with which a person or a group is charged." The chiropractic profession's mission is "HOW" to increase the public knowledge of what chiropractic is, why chiropractic does what it does, and how chiropractic does what it does. The student may ask: "What is the action plan or the strategy of the chiropractic profession to achieve its mission?" Fundamentally, it is to practice exclusively, the chiropractic objective. From a humanitarian point of view, the mission of chiropractic care is to restore the transmission of innate impulses through the practice of its objective (Prin. 27, 28, 29, 31a, 31b).

The short narrative as a mission statement for the chiropractic profession is:

The ***mission*** of chiropractors is the specific task of increasing the awareness of the universal values of chiropractic. Chiropractors accomplish this task by sharing their professional ***vision*** through educating everyone about WHAT chiropractic is, WHY it does what it does, and HOW it does it. In doing so, chiropractors share their professional ***vision*** which is to insure the availability of chiropractic care to everyone. As chiropractors practice the chiropractic ***objective***, (to locate, analyze, and facilitate the correction of vertebral subluxation for an innate-normal transmission of innate impulses), the ***mission*** will allow chiropractic's ***purpose*** to be made manifest, which is to restore the momentum of transmission of innate impulses through the practice of its ***objective***.

ART. 208. INTRODUCTION TO VOLUME 3

Volume 3 consists of the explanation of coordination of activities of body parts and chiropractic's applied science, the practical application of the principles of chiropractic's basic science in analysis. These topics encompass the study of the autonomic nerve system, innate-normal transmission of innate impulses, DIS-EASE, attenuation of the momentum of innate impulses, methods and analysis of vertebral subluxations in accordance with the 33 principles of chiropractic's basic science.

As a basis for Volume 3, Volume 1 explained what is meant by innate-normal, the function of the innate law of living things in the body (Prin. 27). It further explained natural laws and it presented a number of fundamental principles. This was built upon, in Volume 2, which took up the study of cycles.

The 2027 Chiropractic Textbook is an updated systematic presentation regarding the study of chiropractic for classroom use with the curriculum of chiropractic institutions. Its four volumes continually reveal the chiropractic objective, which is derived from the 33 principles of chiropractic's basic science, and how to apply the objective in practice. The articles continue to be numbered from where Volume 2 left off and the method employed is the same.

ART. 209. THE PHYSICAL BRAIN (CENTRAL PROCESSING UNIT)

The physical brain is an organ comprised of nerve tissue located in the cranial cavity. It is utilized by the innate law, which is everywhere in the body, as a centralization control of information/F for the purpose of coordination of activities. It is the central point of coordination. It is the CPU (Central Processing Unit) for the operations of the principle of continuous supply and computation within the living body-computer through innate control (Prin. 33).

The neurons, used by the innate law, centralize innate information/F that has been assembled in the innate field to be conducted through the nerves for coordination of activities. The innate law is intrinsic to all tissue cells of the body. The innate information/F that will be conducted through nerves for coordination of activities originate in the physical brain, which is the central processing unit (CPU) for assemblage and for distribution. It is where innate impulses are continuously coded and computed for coordination of actions of all the parts of the body, if it is possible according to universal laws (Prin. 23, 24). As the brain is an organ, the brain cell is a smaller unit of the brain. The brain cells form the structure of the CPU where the innate law centralizes the innate impulses to be conducted through the nerves for coordination of activities. Metabolically, it is a tissue cell requiring innate information/F, blood, and serum (body chemistry). The innate information/F for metabolism of the tissue cells is innate rays/waves emanating from within the tissue cell. In practice, chiropractic does not address innate rays/waves for metabolism of the tissue cell.

A brain cell is a nerve tissue cell. It is one of the four primary tissues. It has many properties of other tissue cells, having a body and a nucleus. It is called a neuron or a glia. A neuron has a unique architecture as compared to other tissue cells. According to NIH, a neuron has three basic parts: a cell body and two extensions called an axon and a dendrite. Within the body of the cell is a nucleus and other intra-cell particulates (see lexicon) where the cell's activities take place and the cell's genetic material is contained. The axon looks like a long tail and transmits messages from the cell. Dendrites look like the branches of a tree and receive messages from the cell. The glial cells support the neurons in their work; they are called astrocytes and oligodendrocytes.[36]

---

36. https://www.nids.nih.gov/health-information/public-education/brain-basics-life-and-death-neuron#:~:text=A%20%20has%20three%20three%20basic,sends%20messages%20from%20the%20cell (Feb 25, 2025).

Axons bundle forming the spinal cord extending from the brain down through the spinal canal. They ramify, branching to all parts of the body for coordination of actions (Prin. 23, 28). The brain and spinal cord form the central nerve system. The nerves form the peripheral nerve system.

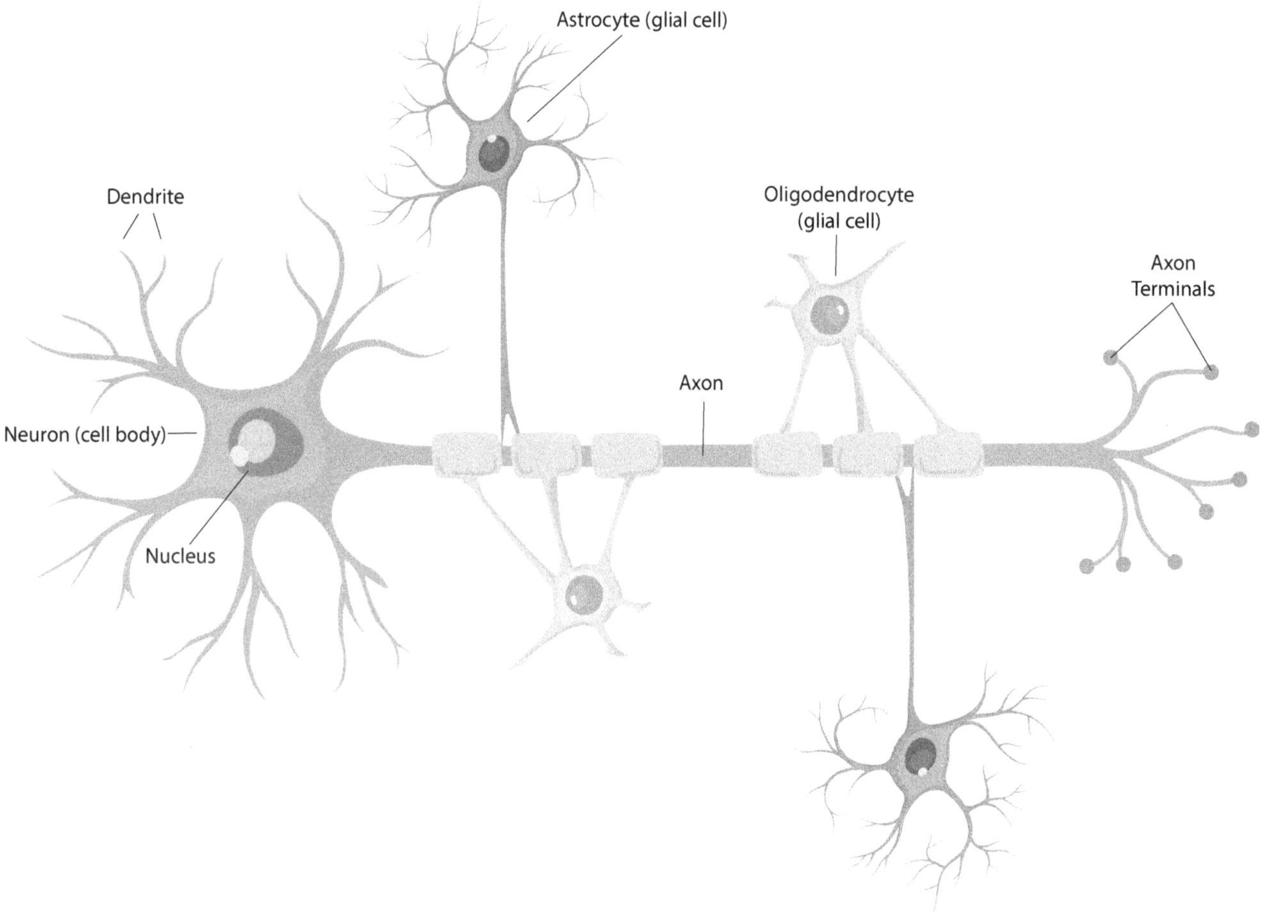

Fig. 29. *This diagram demonstrates the components of the neuron.*

All innate impulses are transmitted to the tissue cells of the body parts for coordination of activities and are sent from the physical brain. All innate rays/waves are radiated from within the tissue cells of the body parts and are for metabolism of the body parts for use in the body (Prin. 23). In practice, chiropractic addresses only the interference in transmission of innate impulses for coordination of activities caused by the vertebral subluxation. This is a very important distinction to make and understand because on it rests the whole purpose of chiropractic.

The physical brain is the control center operated by the innate law for coordination of activities of all the parts of the body. Innate law has no specific location in the body. Therefore, the physical brain is the CPU operated by the innate law to process information/F and codify innate impulses for coordination of actions of all the parts of the body for mutual benefits (Prin. 23). Since the innate law is always 100%/perfect and normal (Prin. 22, 27) there will always be 100%/perfect adaptation and computation if it is possible according to universal laws (Prin. 24).

ART. 210. INNATE FIELD

The innate field is that non-discrete aspect of the body that is utilized by the innate law, as an operating system to adapt, assemble, compute, code, and characterize universal information/F into innate information/F. The innate field is operated by the innate control to compute, assemble innate information/F for use in the body, and for coordination of activities (Prin. 23). It is supplied with innate information/F to function directly from the innate law. It is the operating system of the innate control to govern everything in the body. It is vital and cannot lack ease since it is 100%/perfect and is non-discrete, just like the innate law (Prin. 22). Its location is wherever the innate law is in the body, which is everywhere within the body. Its existence is actual, it is vital, and it is operated by the innate control.

There is no transmission, radiation or oscillation involved in the supply of innate information/F to the innate field by the innate law. There is no necessity, since they both are non-discrete. They are everywhere within the body. For this reason, the innate field always has 100%/perfect innate information/F. It has 100%/perfect function to satisfy the principle of coordination of action (Prin. 32), if it is possible according to universal laws (Prin. 24). It is subject to trauma since it interfaces with the body where the non-material unites with the material and the non-discrete with the discrete through innate information/F (Prin. 10). The innate field is a means by which the interaction between the innate law and the interoperability of all information/F and body functions is achieved in order to be governed. The innate field is the system employed by the innate law, through which it organizes and assembles information/F, thus uniting itself with living E/matter. The innate field must be supplied with sustenance since it interfaces and interacts with E/matter. The innate field is an interface medium that is a field of operations to assemble innate information/F and is located everywhere within all the tissues of the living body. It is the field of computing operations used by the innate law to control, assemble, process, and govern the living body. What happens in any part of the innate field is operated by the innate control. It is the operating system of the innate law for computing everything. Whatever happens in the innate field is simultaneously experienced everywhere in the innate field. It is the field where the computing, characterizing, coding, and assembling of constructive information/F happens, and where the innate control of the innate law governs every process of the living body, without exception. For this reason, the innate field will only operate if it is possible according to universal laws. The innate law-software operating within the innate field is limited by the limitation of E/matter, therefore, the innate field will only operate if it is possible according to universal laws (Prin. 24).

The innate field is where universal information/F is adapted, computed, and coded into innate information/F. For the human body, innate information/F is called innate impulse, trophic impulse/signal, educated impulse, sensory impulse, and innate ray/wave. The innate impulse is transmitted through the efferent nerve system for coordination of activities of all the parts of the body. The trophic impulse/signal is conducted through the afferent nerve system, waved through the innate field to the physical brain for feedback actions of all the body parts. The educated impulse is conducted through the motor nerve system for voluntary actions. The sensory impulse is conducted through the sensory nerve system containing data from the external environment for adaptation to outside conditions. The innate ray/wave is emanated directly from within all the tissue cells of the body for cellular metabolism.

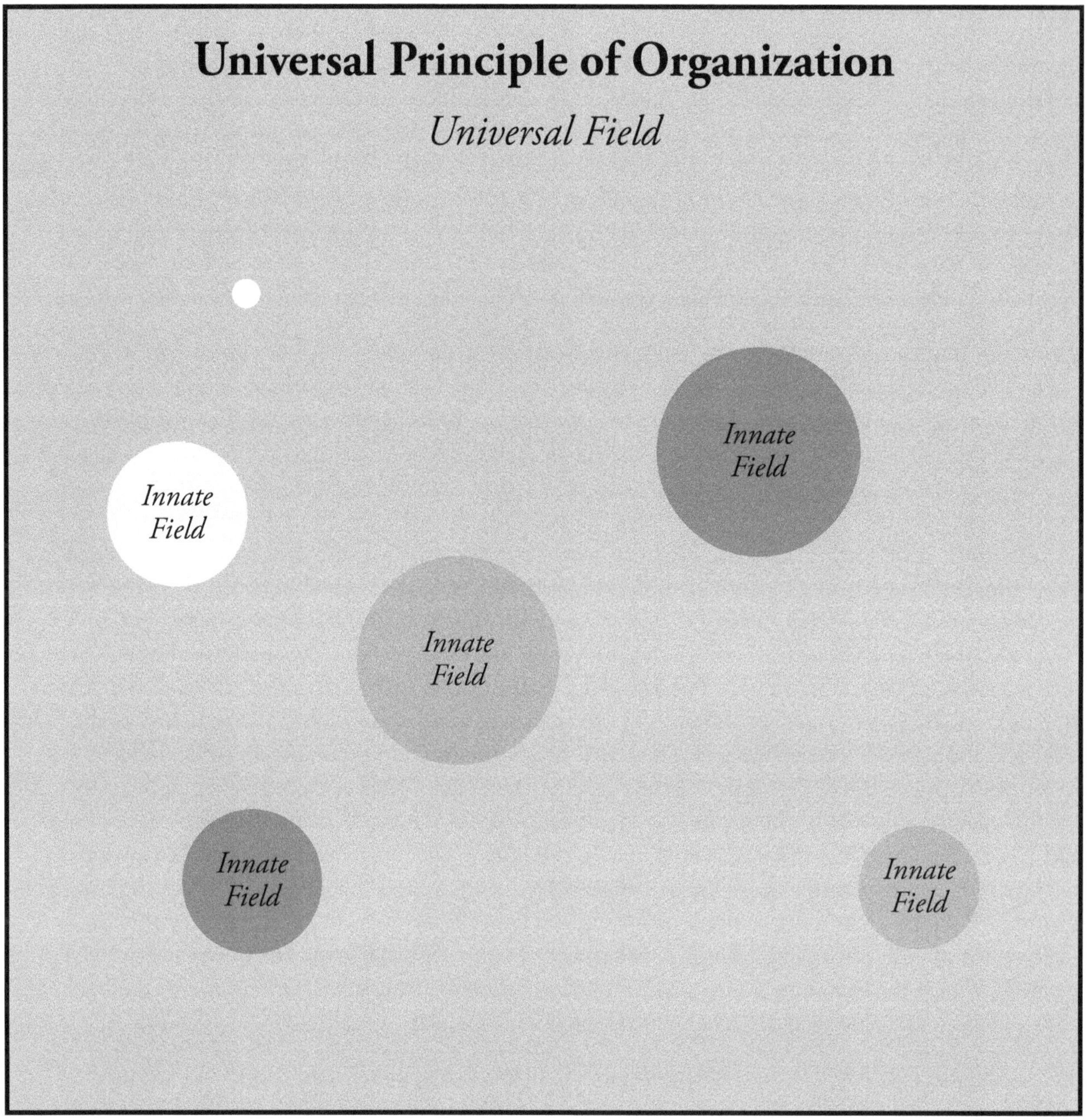

Fig. 30. The box indicates all existence, living and non-living, that is maintained by the universal principle of organization indicated in regular grey. The innate law of living things is a part of and a part from the universal principle of organization. The innate law is an essential extension of the universal principle of organization caused a universal intelligence. It is possible only for living E/matter (and information/F) to be adaptable by the innate law, so as to maintain it alive for a lifetime. The degree of adaptation from the innate law is contingent upon levels of organization of E/matter (Prin. 24). Living things are represented as innate fields within existence under the universal principle of organization; part of it, yet distinct. They are varying shades of grey to suit their level of complexity. They are all still grey. Just a shade of grey adapted according to various states of living E/matter.

REVIEW QUESTIONS FOR ARTICLES 208 - 210

1. What is the study of Volume 3?
2. What is the physical brain anatomically?
3. What is the brain philosophically?
4. What is the necessity of having one central processing unit in the human body?
5. What is the innate field philosophically?
6. Where is the location of the innate field in the body of a living thing?
7. Why is the innate field vital?
8. How does the innate field get its information/F?
9. In what manner are the components of the innate field maintained active?

ART. 211(A). EDUCATED BRAIN

The educated brain is mostly that part of the physical brain used by the innate law of living things, as an organ, for reason, memory, education, conscience, and for voluntary functions. It is supplied with innate impulses for coordination of activities and innate rays/waves for metabolism by the innate law. It is liable to in-coordination as any other tissue, which is always due to vertebral subluxations directly or indirectly (Prin. 31a, 31b), thus it can have in-coordination of action. It is not vital. It is not a vital spot and its location is theoretical. It is most probably within all the cells of the body, but most likely concentrated within the cerebral cortex of the physical brain. It is the chief organ of adaptation to environmental conditions. It is an organ constructed of neurons and happens to be mostly located in the cranium. It is a major organ of adaptation to the outside environment. It is strictly material and as such it expresses information/F (Prin. 13).

As previously mentioned that if you could see the human body as it really is, you would see that it is proportionally as void as intergalactic space. You would see a huge empty void with a few scattered dots and some random electrical discharges. The reason that macroscopic and microscopic properties of particles are similar is because they are both comprised of the same electrons, protons and neutrons. The universe is truly very well organized through and through. And the question arises: What is the nature of this void?

We recognize today that this void is 99.9999% of the physical body.[37] It is just empty space. Is it an emptiness, a nothing, or is it a fullness of some non-material state of information/F? In 1949 B.J. Palmer, D.C. addressed that in his book titled, *"The Bigness of the Fellow Within."*[38] Chiropractic recognizes the fact that the body is 99.9% empty space containing .01% of E/matter. This empty space is actually a non-discrete universal field where the universal principle of organization is organizing information/F to maintain E/matter in existence (Prin. 1).

In the early 2020's, some very interesting research showed that this may be the case. This universal field is a field of all possibilities, a field of infinity, a field of unification. This is literally a field of organization that bespeaks intelligence. This universal field is caused, philosophically speaking, by a universal intelligence. The student may ask, "What causes this universal intelligence?" The answer to that question is found outside the realm of chiropractic philosophy. Chiropractic is a philosophy, a science, and an art.

There is some research that shows that whenever you think, the brain will make a certain chemical as a result of the thought. Any thoughts that you have right now, from your educated brain, are emerging from somewhere through space/time and these thoughts are universal information/F that are adapted and constructed into certain molecules by the innate law. These molecules in the brain are called neuropeptides. "Neuro" because they are in the brain and, "peptides" because when you analyze them, they are protein-like molecules. The way one part of a brain communicates with another part of the brain is not necessarily in English, or any other spoken language, rather it communicates in the language of these neuropeptides.

Neuropeptides are the adapted universal information/F producing body chemistry that are the equivalent of thoughts, feelings, emotions, desires, instincts, drives and ideas. Anytime one has an idea, or concept, or a notion, immediately there is the generation of these neuropeptides in the brain. The neuropeptide is like a messenger molecule, a key that fits into a lock. There are other cells in other parts of the brain

---

37. Sundermier, Ali. "The Particle Physics of You." symmetrymagazine.org/articlethe-particle-physics-of-you?language_content_entity=und (Nov 3,2025).

38. Palmer, B.J., "The Bigness of the Fellow Within" (Vol 22) Davenport, IA: Chiropractic Fountainhead (1949) p. 21

that have receptors to them and the neuropeptides fit into these receptors. That is how the message is delivered/received, and that message is translated into a chemical process in other brain cells. That is how the educated brain cells communicate with each other when you have thoughts.

In the last 40 years, receptors to these neuropeptides have been discovered not just in brain cells but in other parts of the body.

For example, if you look at immune cells (T-cells, B-cells, lymphocytes, monocytes, etc.) which are circulating all over the body (used by the innate law to keep natural resistance balanced), these cells have receptors in them for each of the neuropeptides. Through immune cells, the innate law is literally monitoring the internal dialogues of the body.

Everyone is constantly having thoughts. Thoughts are nothing but conversations with ourselves, and these conversations are monitored by lymphocytes used by the innate law. One cannot have a thought, an emotion, or a desire that escapes the attention of the lymphocytes, the monocytes, the T-cells, the B-cells and all the cells of the immune system.

The 1970's saw a series of important discoveries centering on a new class of minute chemicals called neurotransmitters.[39] These chemicals are part of the structure of neurons that facilitate the transmission of impulses (innate impulse, educated impulse, sensory impulse, trophic impulse/signal). They are conducted innate information/F that act in the body as "communicator molecules", whereby the innate control uses the neurons of the brain to relate coded messages to all the parts of the body using innate impulses for coordination of activities, and body chemistry for cellular metabolism, if it is possible according to universal laws (Prin. 23, 24).

Neurotransmitters make the interaction of information/F and E/matter far more mobile and flowing than ever before. They aid the understanding of how they fill the gap that apparently separates mind and body, one of the deepest mysteries that mankind has faced since the beginning of self-knowledge. The previous volumes stated that educated intelligence grows and evolves overtime (personally and collectively).

Let us review some of the known evolutionary process of educated intelligence, which is the activity of the educated brain:

In 1973, it seemed that the innate law was out of necessity running only two neurotransmitters: one for activating a distant cell, such as a muscle, and the other to slow down the activity, (acetylcholine and norepinephrine, respectively).

Neurotransmitters are the "go" and "stop" of the central nerve system. They are like binary numbers "0" and "1", that can be flipped "on" and "off" according to the parameters of the tissue cells (Prin. 33). It is the property that can be set to one of at least two states ("1" ~~ "0" or "0" ~~ "1"). This observation specifies the following computation: if the neurotransmitter is "1" flip it to "0", if "0" flip it to "1". The reason a computer can perform this computation is because it has been copied from what already exist in principles. It is an exact copy of what is being computed within the human body by the innate law. In Volume 1, the property of copy-ability was introduced, whereas we cannot give that which we do not have to have. This literally means that anything that is to be constructed must have the property of copy-ability because the universe is forever 100% complete (Prin. 5). The properties of interoperability, of adaptability, of copyability and flipability are universal properties.

---

39. López-Muñoz, F, Alamo, C, "Historical Evolution of the Neurotransmission Concept." Journal of Neural Transmission, 2009 May; 116:515-33

Neurotransmitters were considered revolutionary at the time because they empirically proved that impulses (innate, trophic, educated, sensory) transmitted from one neuron to the next were electrical, AND chemical in nature. They were chemo-electric and organized by the innate law in such a way as to communicate information/F from one neuron to the other. As molecular biologists around the world began to investigate more deeply this finding, numerous neurotransmitters were discovered.

By mid 1980's, barely 10 years after the original breakthrough, more than 50 neurotransmitters and neuropeptides were known. In 2024, over 100 are known. All of them can be manufactured on either side of the synapses between neurons, and once they cross the synapses, all of them can be received by the receptor cells on the other side, and vice-versa. This implies an incredible flexibility of interoperability to communicate from cell to cell, all organized under innate control. As many as ten trillion connections are possible at any given moment. This reveals an amazing organization that bespeaks intelligence. In chiropractic this intelligence is demonstrated through "The Universal Diagram of Cycles" (*See Fig. 5*). It is an innate bioelectric chemical information/F computing feedback loop system continually processed by the innate control. This feedback loop is comprised of efferent and afferent nerves, and it is applicable to every part of the body for coordination of actions of those parts for mutual benefit, thus to benefit the whole body (Prin. 23). This brought about many frustrating complications for researchers but for our purpose as chiropractors it once again demonstrates that the body cannot be understood without the missing ingredient of intelligence.

The discovery by the Palmers in the early 1900's, of this non-material field of information/F adapted by the innate law of living things is a built-in feature designed to be part of all the E/matter of our bodies. Organization bespeaks intelligence. It is a universal intelligence that causes and constructs a universal principle of organization in order to continually organize information/F giving properties and actions to all E/matter, thereby maintaining it in existence (Prin. 1). An essential extension of this universal organizing principle is the innate law of living things, whose function is to adapt higher and more complex levels and states of E/matter to maintain it alive for a while if it is possible according to universal laws (Prin. 20, 22, 23, 24).

In his greater modification of the Safety Pin Cycle, B.J. Palmer, D.C. showed us that the innate law permeates every tissue cell of the human body.[40] Brain cells send innate impulses through neuro-synaptic efferent transmission of the nerve system and those innate impulses are received by the body part receptor for coordination of activities. After the innate impulses are received by the receptor body part, the innate law operating that receptor part decodes the innate impulses. It further processes the receptor cell sending trophic impulses/signals through neuro-synaptic afferent transmission of the nerve system to its cell body, waving the signals through the innate field, back to brain cells for decoding and interpretation by instantaneous integral innate processing. The reason it happens this way is because we can only construct that which has the properties of copy-ability and universality. We can construct computers with software and hardware that process computation using cybernetic feedback loop systems because of the properties of copyability and universality of the human body. In other words what we construct is a copy of what already exists. In 21st century terms, all the Lego pieces already exist and are maintained in existence through being organized by the universal principle of organization and the innate law of living things (Prin. 5, 22). All we are required to do is to have a working knowledge of these principles and apply them in practice.

For example, the innate law codes, computes, and processes information/F of immune cells to make the same body chemistry or the same neuropeptides that the brain makes when you use it to think. It is

40. Stephenson, R.W., "Chiropractic Text Book." (Vol XIV) Davenport, IA: The Palmer School of Chiropractic. (1948) p. 9,11

accomplished through the property of interoperability allowing the immune cells to be used as thinking cells because they produce the exact same chemicals that the educated brain makes when it thinks.

As the educated brain evolved, the word neuropeptide became an obsolete word. It is no longer being used because the peptide is not confined to the physical brain since it can be found in other parts of the body. An alternate term that was used was immuno-modulators, because these chemicals, which are the equivalent of thoughts, are processed by the innate law to modulate the activity of the immune system. That alternate term becomes obsolete because when we start examining the human body looking for these chemicals, they are everywhere. This demonstrates the evolutionary adaptability that the educated brain continually undergoes. Our understanding grows over time. It has personal values. On the other hand, the principles of chiropractic's basic science have universal values and are absolute, immutable and unchangeable. They can only be refined as our understanding grows through the evolutionary process of our educated intelligence. It is our understanding of the innate law through observation and research that continually grows over time (Prin. 6).

Another example is that stomach cells also make the same peptides that the brain makes when you use it to think and respond to them. It is also true of gut cells, lung cells, heart cells, skin cells, and kidney cells; they all make the same peptides and respond to the same peptides. This is due to the counterfactual property of interoperability of information/F from the innate law studied in Volume 1.

Now when you say, I have a gut feeling about such and such, you're not speaking metaphorically at all, you're speaking very literally because your gut cells make the exact same chemicals than the brain cells would if it were having those thoughts. In fact, the gut feeling may be a little more accurate because the gut has not evolved to the stage of self-doubt, which neurons perhaps have.

The same story is true with heart cells. When you say, I have a sad heart or my heart is bursting with love and joy, you are speaking literally because, under innate control, the heart makes those chemicals which are the equivalent of those thoughts. In fact, we have a thinking body. Every cell of the human body is a thinking cell. The physical brain only appears to be the thinking organ of the body.

Intelligence has escaped the confines of the brain. Stephenson's stated in 1927 that "we must never conceive of it (educated brain) as a Power which creates thoughts or as a thing that can govern the body. It is merely a piece of flesh, just as helpless in this matter as a steak in the butcher's window… The educated brain is used by Innate to receive precepts concerning the environment of the body."[41]

Educated intelligence was equated with the brain. However, with all these new findings, it can no longer be equated. Educated intelligence has escaped the confines of the physical brain and it is in every cell of our body. Every cell of our body is in fact an intelligent cell, a thinking cell. All the cells in the body think simultaneously through the "innate law of the cell." There is no hierarchy that the brain thinks first, hypothalamus thinks second, then the heart thinks. It is not that way at all.

For example, imagine having the thought or idea that one is thirsty and they need water. The innate law will adapt and process my brain cells to make a chemical called angiotensin-2. That chemical influences behavior in such a way that one will start looking for a water bottle or start asking somebody where one may get some water. Through innate control, the hypothalamus also makes a chemical called angiotensin-2, which causes the secretion of another hormone called ADH. This encourages the body to hold on to water, but at the same time heart cells make angiotensin-2, heart cell hold on to water, and kidney cells make angiotensin-2, so one doesn't lose water in the urine. Skin cells make angiotensin-2 because they are dehydrating. The idea one is thirsty does not emerge first in the physical brain. It is

41. Stephenson, R.W., "Chiropractic Text Book." (Vol XIV) Davenport, IA: The Palmer School of Chiropractic. (1948) p. 13-15

simultaneously everywhere in the entire body. The innate law processes each cell at the same time. It is called 100%/instantaneous integral adaptation. The educated brain is everywhere in the body despite the common belief that thoughts are first generated in the physical brain. It is all about an integral process of body chemistry and of information/F that is adapted and organized by the innate law. This is due to interoperability which is a characteristic of the activity of the innate law in the innate field.

This is a new paradigm which says that the ideas, which are organized innate information/F, are not even confined to our bodies for they are everywhere in all of space and time, all at the same time, we have a thinking body governed by the innate law. This thinking body is part of a thinking universe comprised of a universal principle of organization that organizes universal information/F initiated by a universal intelligence. This universal principle of organization is the initial condition of chiropractic's basic science (Prin. 1).

There is enough data that are emerging, that show that, ideas, notions, and thoughts are field phenomena emerging from a universal field of information/F, organized by the universal principle of organization, which is a field of all possibilities and potentialities. This is literally a field. Chiropractic is about what is possible according to universal laws (Prin. 24). We just did not know that in 1927. D.D., B.J., and Stephenson were visionaries beyond our ability to understand. Yet, they forged forward with what their educated brain knew at the time, and carried on.

Today when we analyze a field of all possibilities, we cannot limit ourselves to space or time. If you tickle the electromagnetic field in one place, the whole field is affected.

This model of educated intelligence employing the educated brain, which is everywhere in the body, precedes physical manifestations. There is an innate law that causes both the mind and the body to emerge. Many clinical studies hold this to be true, which is verifying and validating the principles of chiropractic's basic science.[42]

The discovery of neuro-transmitters, neuropeptides, neuro-modulators and messenger molecules of all kinds has vastly extended our concept and understanding of biological organization. If every cell has endless number of messages it can send and receive, governed by the innate law, it is also clear that only a small fraction is activated at one time for each cell. The question arises,

"What controls the messengers and the countless changes in body chemistry?" The innate law of living things governs all tissue cells of the body through adapting, computing, processing, and coding universal information/F into innate information/F for use in the body and for coordination of all the parts of the body for mutual benefit (Prin. 20, 23).

It is an interesting question for the people of the world today. In a chemistry lab, it may appear that reactions will run automatically as soon as the experiment starts, yet something has to allow the chemicals to reorganize and not merely a matter of mixing one chemical with another.

The world has struggled to apply this fact to the human body. In chiropractic, there are thousands of chemicals at the disposal of the innate law within the field of a single cell. The innate law must adapt information/F to produce the appropriate chemicals, mix them together and analyze the results. The innate law is computing thousands of data processes to reorganize new molecules out of basically a handful of elements: carbon, oxygen, hydrogen and nitrogen. To do that requires organization, and organization bespeaks intelligence, which is the causality of the innate law of living things.

---

42. Wong, L, Cleland, C.E., et al. "On the Roles of Function and Selection in Evolving Systems." PNAS Vol. 120, No. 43 (2023) doi: 10.1073.2310223120

So, via the story of neuropeptides, the dramatic shift in worldview is observed pointing toward chiropractic philosophy. Chiropractic was so far ahead of its time in the 1920's having formulated 33 principles that revealed organization bespeaking intelligence. In the 2020's, the purpose of chiropractic with its objective, and the vision of chiropractors including their professional mission, points to an evolutionary approach to life with all that it entails.

For the first time in the history of the world, the innate law of living things has a visible scaffold to stand upon a solid platform. Before this, the communities of the world declared that human beings were physical machines that had somehow learned to think. Now it dawns on many that we are non-discrete bits of innate information/F that have been organized by the innate law into a physical machine. D.D. Palmer wrote in his 1910 book, *The Adjustor* that, "We are Intelligence expressing itself through matter."[43]

Today we have the Quantum Bio-Cybernetic-Mental feedback loop, which shows how brain cells communicate with tissue cells.[44] B.J. Palmer called it "The Safety Pin Cycle." The world later came about this realization around the 1990's when some research that was done at Ohio State University clearly demonstrated again that these peptides are also produced in other parts of the human body, showing that the mind has escaped the confinement of the brain and that we have, in reality, a "thinking" body and that thoughts do not emerge in the brain first but in the entire body all at once. This research supports the chiropractic understanding of bio-electric impulses that were measured in 1952 by the Palmer Clinic using the Electroencephaloneuromentypograph.[45] In chiropractic, we do not seek to alter the innate law, neither do we seek to alter the energy/matter. What we deal with is the link between the two which is called information/force. This is reminiscent of B.J.'s famous pun, "Christian Scientists always mind, never matter; Medical Doctors always matter, never mind."

In the early 1950's, Francis Crick and James Watson cracked open the genetic code and they found that the only thing that the genes do is transmit information/F, not energy, not matter, only information/F[46]. That is what chiropractic is all about, the normal transmission of conducted innate information/F (innate impulse) that can be interfered with by vertebral subluxations (Prin. 31a).

The educated brain is an organ used by the innate law for several specific purposes, just as the liver or stomach are used for certain purposes. The educated brain is constructed of living E/matter, and therefore it has limitations (Prin. 24). A multitude of causes can create breakdowns in the following processes due to the limitations of E/Matter: thinking, intuition, instinct, intellectual processing of computation, reasoning, memory storage and retrieval, environmental perceptions and assessments, modification of tinctured innate impulses into educated impulses, and the voluntary actions pertaining to the will. The property of the educated brain to perceive external conditions is necessary for the innate law to receive percepts from the environment of the body, for its comfort and welfare. The innate law uses the educated brain to store percepts through a physiological reconstruction of its constant change in structure. The accumulation of percepts, including data, is formed into knowledge and is what constitutes education. At birth, educated intelligence is 0% evolving over time. At death educated intelligence has reached its maximum of 100%, because this person's educated intelligence will cease to develop.

---

43. Palmer, D.D., editior B.J.Palmer. " The Chiropractic Adjuster." Davenport, IA: The Palmer School of Chiropractic. (1921) p.772

44. Funk, Richard H.W., "Understanding the Feedback Loops Between Energy, Matter, and Life." Front.Biosci. (Elite Ed.) 2022, 14(4)29. doi: 10.310083/j.fbe1404029

45. Palmer, B.J., "Chiropractic Clinical Controlled Research." Davenport, IA: Chiropractic Fountain Head. (1951) p. 219-220

46. Tamura, Koji. "The Genetic Code: Francis Crick's Legacy and Beyond" Life 2016; 6(3):36 doi: 10.3390/life6030036

Chiropractic only addresses one cause: vertebral subluxation, which interferes with the momentum of transmission of innate impulses for coordination of activities of body parts (Prin. 23, 30, 31a). Chiropractic is the philosophy, the science, and the art whose objective is to locate, analyze and facilitate the correction of vertebral subluxations for an innate-normal transmission of innate impulses in accordance to the principles of its basic science. Nothing more. Nothing less. Nothing else (*See Art. 2,4)* (Prin. 29, 30, 31a, 31b).

ART. 211 (B). VOLUNTARY ACTIONS

The "tincturing" of innate impulses to modify them into educated impulses for voluntary actions is a capability of the educated brain of the individual made possible by the counterfactual property of copy-ability which imbues a specific character of their resolve to an innate impulse that transforms it into an educated impulse to perform a certain voluntary act. The original innate impulse is an adapted, computerized, characterized, and coded universal information/F by the innate law; then it is imbued by the educated brain, with a specific new character, and transformed into an educated impulse for voluntary actions. When an innate impulse goes through the educated brain, it can be tinctured by educated intelligence through volition, for modification into an educated impulse for a voluntary act.

The educated brain is an organ that possesses a capability to utilize educated intelligence, the learned versatility that can modify innate impulses to carry out voluntary actions. The educated brain has the ability to recode, or tincture, innate impulses through recharacterization into a thought, or educated impulse. Information/F has the counterfactual property of copy-ability and, therefore can be recoded. Universal information/F can be adapted and recoded into innate information/F by the perfect innate law for use the body (Prin. 23). Innate information/F can also be tinctured, and recoded by the less than perfect educated intelligence, due to limitation of E/matter of the educated brain (Prin. 24) for conscious activities.

Note: The student is reminded that the universal principle of organization is the initial condition of chiropractic's basic science. It is the fundamental principle that continually organizes information/F to provide properties and actions to all E/matter to maintain it in existence. Information/F is then adapted by the innate law, which is an essential extension of the universal principle of organization, into innate impulses for coordination of activities of all the parts of the living body, or are adapted into innate rays/waves for metabolism for all the cells of the body (Prin. 23). Innate impulses can then be tinctured and modified into educated impulses by the individual's resolve, utilizing his/her educated intelligence, which is the capability of the educated brain to function for voluntary actions. Ultimately, it is the innate law that governs all processes of the body, including educated impulses from the educated brain tinctured by the resolve of the individual's educated intelligence.

ART. 212. THE SPINAL CORD

The spinal cord is a bundle of nerve axons, which is used by the innate law to conduct innate information/F to and from the physical brain. The spinal cord is a continuation of the brain stem and is part of the central nerve system. It is the main conductor of innate impulses to the peripheral nerves for coordination of activities of all the parts of the body. Its branches, the spinal nerves, emit through the inter-vertebral foramina and ramify to all parts of the body. While all tissue cells have innate rays/waves for metabolism, along with body chemistry from the serous circulation, the coordinative action of all the parts of the body is dependent upon innate impulses, which must arrive via the spinal cord in a timely manner (Prin. 6). This is accounted for through clinical findings and laboratory experiments that all the parts of the body are subject to in-coordination, if the transmitting neurons of the spinal cord or spinal nerve are lacking ease (DIS-EASE) due to impingements caused by vertebral subluxations.[47] Everything in the body depends upon everything else for coordination of activities. It is all about body chemistry and information/F that are adapted and organized by the innate law. Therefore, it is essential that all the parts of the body have an innate-normal transmission of innate impulses (without interference from vertebral subluxations), and that the tissue cell maintains an innate-normal vitality through the soundness of its metabolism.

ART. 213. SPINAL NERVES

Spinal nerves are the branches from the spinal cord, which leave the neural canal via the inter-vertebral foramina on both sides of the spine.There is a pair of nerves located superiorly to each vertebra of the spinal column. There are 31 pairs of spinal nerves comprised of both efferent and afferent axons. Each pair is said arbitrarily to belong to the vertebra below it.

Efferent nerves are used for transmission of conducted innate information/F from the physical brain-CPU to the body-part-receptor for coordination of activities. The word, efferent, indicates direction. Merriam-Webster Dictionary defines *efferent* as "conveying nervous impulses to an effector." This word is derived from Latin, effere, which means to "carry outward." The route is from physical brain cell to tissue cell, from CPU to receptor.

Efferent nerves are transmitters of innate impulses. They begin in the physical brain leading out through the spinal cord and emitting to all the parts of the body. Coordination of action of body parts would not be possible without such nerve supply.

Afferent nerves are used for transmission of conducted information/F (trophic impulses/signals) from body-part-receptor to the physical brain-CPU, conveying feedback, for coordination of activities. The word, afferent, also indicates direction. The Merriam-Webster Dictionary defines *afferent* as "conveying impulses toward the central nervous system." This word is derived from Latin, affere, which means to "carry inward." The route is from tissue cell to physical brain cell, from receptor to CPU.

Afferent nerves are transmitters of trophic impulses/signals and begin in the body-part-receptor and lead to the physical brain-CPU for feedback regarding coordination of activities. Coordination of action of body parts would not be possible without such information feedback. Feedback must always be true in order to be valid feedback, whether from normal functions or from abnormal functions, for coordination of activities. This means that vertebral subluxations cannot interfere with transmission of feedback. This is corroborated and verified anatomically as vertebral subluxations cannot impinge upon afferent nerve cells bodies since they run outside the spinal nerves waving the trophic impulse/signal through the innate field to the physical brain (not to be confused with the afferent nerves of the special sense cycle).

Only efferent nerves can be impinged by vertebral subluxations for coordination of activities.

47. Sharpless, S.K., "Susceptibility of Spinal Nerve Roots to Compression Block." DHEW Publication (NIH) 767-998, (1975)

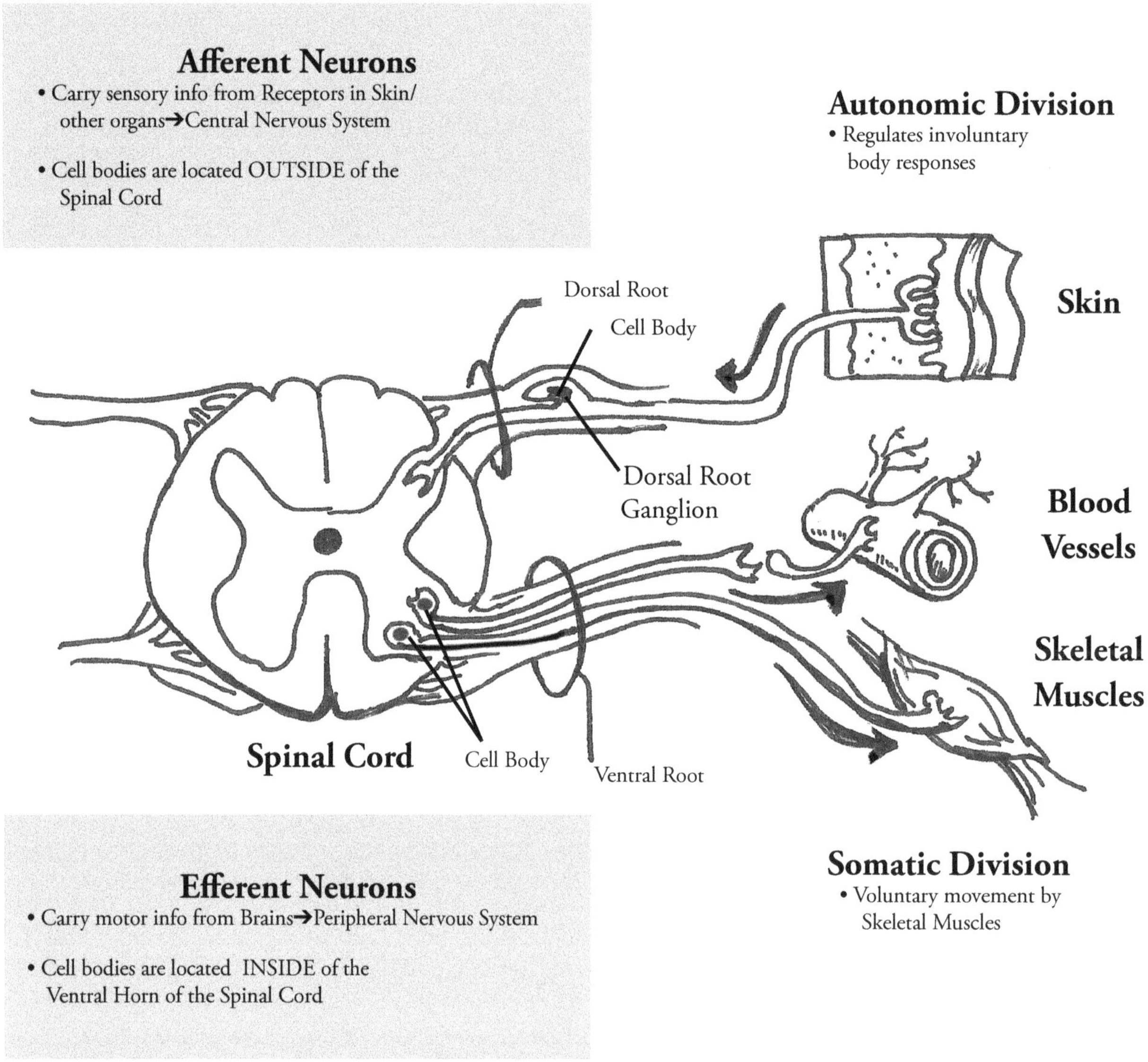

Fig. 31. Diagram demonstrating efferent nerves where the cell bodies are located inside the ventral horn of the spinal cord and subject to impingement by vertebral subluxations; and afferent nerves where the cell bodies are located outside of the spinal cord and are notsubject to impingement by vertebral subluxation.

A nerve is a bundle of axon fibers. An axon is a very minute filament that is part of the neuron, the function of which is to transmit the innate information/F from the brain to the tissue cell of the body part (efferent innate impulse), and from the body part back to the brain as feedback (afferent trophic impulse/signal). When a nerve is impinged, it means that one or more of the axons are impinged and there is lack of ease from these axons. According to S.K. Sharpless, regarding the function of a nerve, "A pressure of only 10mm Hg on a nerve produced a significant conduction block, the potential falling to 60% of its initial value in 15 minutes and to half its initial value in 30 minutes."[48] The function of nerves is to transmit innate information/F. A nerve is a cable-like structure that conducts innate information/F from brain cell to tissue cell and from tissue cell to brain cell. A nerve can only be impinged on the efferent side of the cycle due to the fact that afferent nerves do not have axons, they have dendrites with the neuron cell body outside the spinal cord.

48. Sharpless, S.K., "Susceptibility of Spinal Nerve Roots to Compression Block." DHEW Publication (NIH) 767-998, (1975)

ART. 214. THE PERIPHERY

Periphery is the term used to indicate the tissues at the end of efferent nerves (axons), or at the beginning of afferent nerves (dendrites). It is the tissue, of the body part, that is supplied with innate impulses for coordination of activities. Nerve tissue itself may be periphery.

The physical brain is the central processing unit (CPU) for coordination of activities. The system of transmission of conducted innate information/F for coordination of activities is comprised of the spinal cord, spinal nerves, cranial nerves, and the visceral nerves, and the tissue of the body parts are the periphery. The "physical triunity" is the physical representation of the triune of existence (Prin. 4). Information/F is organized by the organizing principle and is the link between the organizing principle and E/matter (Prin. 10). In the living body, the physical representation is the "physical brain" and the "physical body part" and the "link" between them is innate information/F.

The spinal nerves, in whole bundles, divide into superficial and deep branches. The superficial branches divide and supply the superficial tissues. The branches that supply the deeper tissues transmit conducted innate information/F from the physical brain to the body parts efferently for coordination of activities. All parts of the body are supplied with innate impulses by certain nerves and their branches from the spinal column. Each pair of spinal nerves has a definite division to supply innate impulses to all parts of the body.

Note: At the time of the updating, writing and publishing of this textbook, the author is well aware that new information will be available in the future that is not known yet. Since its discovery, chiropractic has not stood still and will continue to evolve according to new formulated knowledge. What is immutable, absolute, and constant, are the 33 principles of chiropractic's basic science. These principles are unchangeable, however, they can be refined.

Before we continue any further it is important to interject at this time some necessary review regarding chiropractic philosophy, science and art.

ART. 215. PRACTICAL IMPLICATIONS OF APPLYING THE INSTRUCTIVE INFORMATION OF THE 33 PRINICPLES OF CHIROPRACTIC'S BASIC SCIENCE AND THEIR PHILOSOPHICAL EXPLANATIONS

What are the instructions provided by the 33 principles of chiropractic's basic science?

First of all, the initial condition of chiropractic's basic science is its fundamental principle, "A universal principle of organization is continually supplying properties and actions to all E/matter, thus maintaining it in existence." It is called the major premise (Prin. 1). This is the starting point of chiropractic's basic science. It is the first principle that initiates the foundational platform upon which the entire structure of chiropractic is constructed. Its function is to organize information/F. Since organization bespeaks intelligence, chiropractic philosophy asserts that the universal principle of organization has been designed by a universal intelligence.

The universal principle of organization is intrinsic to every particle of E/matter providing it with all of its properties and actions through the organizing information/F. It is manifested by motion (Prin. 14) and is called existence (Prin. 1). The innate law of living things, a distinct process of this organizing principle, keeps alive a specific portion of E/matter for a lifetime through adaptation (Prin. 20) and it is an essential extension of the universal principle of organization. In the living body, the function of an inborn and 100%/perfect innate law is to adapt universal information/F and E/matter in a viable manner (Prin. 21, 23). The organization of the body of living things points to centralization, or compliance functions for coordination of activities. In the human body this center of control is the physical brain. The innate law governs and operates every living cell using the physical brain in order to centralize and distribute conducted information/F via the spinal cord through the spinal column to control coordination of activities of body parts utilizing the nerve trunks emanating from the spinal cord and passing through the inter-vertebral foramina to the nerve branches that supply to all parts of the body (Prin. 28). Perfect adaptation from the innate control, for coordination of activities, depends upon the adaptability of the universal elements of that particular body. Perfect adaptation, for coordination of activities, requires complete control, if that is possible without breaking a universal law (Prin. 24). This perfect adaptation will satisfy the principle of coordination (Prin. 32). Interference with the transmission (Prin. 29) of innate impulses will bring about a lack of ease (Prin. 30) of the neuron-transmitters and will violate the principle of coordination (Prin. 32). Lack of ease is never due to any imperfection of the innate law, because the innate law is always 100%/perfect (Prin. 22), and continuously adapts 100%/perfect information/F (Prin. 27, 33). Lack of ease is due to interference with the momentum of transmission of conducted innate information/F through or over the nerves for coordination of activities (Prin. 29). Since the spinal column is the only segmented structure of bone through which the nerve trunks pass, and there is the possibility of the displacement of these segments, changing the size and shape of the inter-vertebral foramina, it is possible for vertebral subluxations to occur. If a vertebral subluxation does occur, it will cause an interference with the momentum of transmission of conducted innate information/F (Prin. 31a). Lack of ease of transmitting neurons alters the momentum of transmission of conducted innate information/F and will cause in-coordination of activities (Prin. 30). Chiropractic is a science which consists of having a working scientific knowledge of this cause of lack of ease of specific neurons which then alters the momentum of the transmission of the conducted innate information/F (Prin. 30, 31a). The application of these basic principles of chiropractic's basic science solves a specific humanitarian problem, the "vertebral subluxation."

In practice, a specific adjustic thrust is introduced into the vertebral segment involved to facilitate the process of a vertebral adjustment by the innate law (Prin. 31b), thereby removing the interference of the transmission of conducted innate information/F (Prin. 29). The correction of vertebral subluxation does not add or subtract any material to the body, but simply allows the restoration of transmission of innate impulses back to innate-normal which would have been present had there been no interference (Prin. 31b). In this manner, the principle of coordination is fulfilled and satisfied (Prin. 32). Chiropractic includes the study of living things, specifically that of the vertebrate in particular. At the present time the adjustic thrust is confined to the human spine and the spines of a few domestic animals in order to bring about coordination of actions of all the parts of that living body (Prin. 32).

Our study for the application of the principles of chiropractic's basic science, with the exception of the fundamentals, is mainly concerned with the innate law of living things (Prin. 20). The innate law specifically adapts universal information/F and E/matter for use in the body, so that all parts of the body will have coordination of activities (Prin. 23) within limitations of E/matter (Prin. 24). The application of those principles is also concerned with the interference in the transmission of conducted innate information/F, called innate impulses (Prin. 28, 29), caused by vertebral subluxations (Prin. 31a). The specific adjustic thrust facilitates of the correction of the vertebral subluxation by the innate law (Prin. 31b) which satisfies the principle of coordination (Prin. 32). The instructions of those principles provide information to chiropractors to maintain an awareness of whether or not they practice the chiropractic objective. The principles of chiropractic's basic science are a ***G***uiding ***P***rinciple ***S***teering ***S***ystem (GPSS) to help chiropractors to stay on course and not deviate toward metaphysics or therapeutics.

REVIEW QUESTIONS FOR ARTICLES 211 - 215

1. What is educated brain, philosophically?
2. Why is educated brain not a vital spot?
3. How does educated brain get its innate impulses?
4. What distinguishes organisms with highly developed educated brains from others not so well developed?
5. Can educated brain rule the body?
6. What is the spinal cord, anatomically?
7. What is the relationship between the spinal cord and the coordination of activities of all the parts of the living body?
8. What are the spinal nerves, anatomically?
9. How are the spinal nerves classified and named in chiropractic?
10. When impingement occurs are all the axons necessarily affected?
11. Anatomically, is a nerve one axon or a bundle of axons?
12. What is periphery?
13. What is the initial condition of chiropractic's basic science?
14. In practice, which principles of chiropractic's basic science are mainly applied?
15. What is called the GPSS of chiropractic?

The student must understand that chiropractic was discovered at a time when the medical model ruled almost everything that had to do with the human body. This 5000 year old model was the prevalent conception in those days. Therefore, it is understandable that D.D. Palmer's first few students were well intended medical doctors who wanted to add something more to their repertoire to get sick people well. In the early days, both, D.D. and B.J. claimed that chiropractic could get sick people well, much more effectively and less costly than medicine via the correction of vertebral subluxations through specific adjustments of vertebral subluxations. One of the early methods to be used by the chiropractor to find vertebral subluxations was the Meric System. The Meric System is a nerve chart depicting a simple diagram of the brain, the spinal vertebrae and spinal nerves that innervate organs, glands, muscles and vessels. It was used by chiropractors to trace the nerve involved in the symptomatic body part to the location of the specific subluxated vertebra to deliver an adjustic thrust. The Meric System was divided into superior meric system and inferior meric system, the latter of which was further developed into zones and meres.[49] As of 2025 chiropractic is only 130 years old, which means that chiropractic is comparatively very young. Chiropractic has not stood still since its discovery in 1895. It has been developed and continues to grow as we construct new working knowledge from the new information available today. Chiropractic has evolved from getting sick people well, SOMETIMES, through the correction of vertebral subluxations --- to restoring the transmission of innate impulses (Prin. 29), to innate-normal (Prin. 27), for coordination of activities of body parts (Prin. 32), ALL THE TIME, through facilitating the correction of vertebral subluxations by the innate law (Prin. 31a, 31b). The new chiropractic model is constructed on the rock-solid foundational platform comprised of the 33 principles of chiropractic's basic science. Chiropractic's basic science directs us to apply those principles to solve a universal humanitarian problem namely, the vertebral subluxation, through facilitating the process of a vertebral adjustment by the innate law, for an innate-normal transmission of innate impulses.

Considering all that we know and have witnessed as a profession for more than a century, chiropractic experienced a remarkable small start. Yet, every new discovery begins with a small step... a falling fruit for gravity, a lightning spark for electricity, a protruding bump on a spine for chiropractic.

The movement for chiropractic to be further developed continues. This is encouraging, in that any small step we take to understand chiropractic better is productive. A simple resolve to daily read and re-read something within all the Blue Books, the Green Books, including Stephenson's 1927 text, can turn out to be plentiful, if not monumental. Most importantly, the chiropractors can derive encouragement if they continually maintain a learner's mind with an ever-growing desire to continue to be a chiropractic student for their entire career. As we move along the path provided by the new chiropractic model, we will catch up with how amazing chiropractic is.

In the 1970s it was mentioned within Reggie Gold's fictive obituary, in his story of "The Valley of the Blind," that he was the last living chiropractor.[50] Based on that, one can imagine at the gates of heaven, the angel asks Reggie: "Did you accomplish your task?" "Yes, all is done," he replied. "I have another question Reggie", said the angel. "Has the whole world heard of chiropractic?" "No" said Reggie. The angel asked, "Then what is your plan?" Reggie said, "I have left a few objective chiropractors to carry on the task and change the whole world, because as they focus on changing the world they will realize that everything else just Mickey Mouse." The angel looks at Reggie and asked: "What is your plan B?"

---

49. Hynes, R.J.R., Callender A.K. "Technique in the Classroom at Palmer College of Chiropractic: A history of art in chiropractic." J Chirophuman 2008; 15:55-66

50."The Triune of Life: Reggie Gold's Philosophical Legacy." Senzon, Simon (ed.) Asheville, NC: The Institute Chiropractic. (2022) p.xix-xx

The answer to that question is that there is no plan B. The practice of the chiropractic objective will change the world through objective chiropractors like you and me. Let us together, without condemnation, continue to carry on.

ART. 216. CHIROPRACTIC IS ALWAYS AT CAUSE

Chiropractic is always at cause because according to the 33 principles of chiropractic's basic science, it is concerned with only one function which is a perfect and normal function. It is the function of the non-discrete innate law of living things to govern through adaptation everything in the body (Prin. 20, 23), with 100%/perfect control (Prin. 22) according to universal laws (Prin. 24). The innate law is absolute normal and its function is absolute normal (Prin. 27). It is called innate-normal. Chiropractic does not concern itself with the functions of the discrete body. Chiropractic addresses exclusively the vertebral subluxation, which is the cause of interference in the momentum of transmission of innate impulses (Prin. 29, 31a) due to limitation of E/matter (Prin. 24), which violates the principle of coordination (Prin. 32). Chiropractic never addresses effects. Chiropractic's only purpose is only the facilitation of the correction of the cause of interference of the momentum of transmission of innate impulses for coordination of activities, which is the vertebral subluxation.

ART. 217. CONFIRMATION OF CHIROPRACTIC BEING AT CAUSE THROUGH THE PRINCIPLE OF CONTINUOUS SUPPLY AND COMPUTATION (PRIN. 33)

The principle of continuous supply and computation describes an infinite continuous supply of universal information/F to all E/matter to maintain it in existence. The body is a living universal computer that is adapted and processed by the innate law which is its complete 100%/perfect software that never needs updates. The coordination of activities of its parts requires an innate field, which is the operating system that is located all over the body, where the innate law adapts, computes, processes, and assembles conducted innate information/F. The physical brain is the central processing unit (CPU) for coordination of activities. The processors of the CPU are the brain cells and the transmitters of innate impulses are the nerve cells. Chiropractic is not directly concerned with the receptors, namely the tissue cells of the body parts receiving the innate impulses from the transmitters. Chiropractic remains at cause not effect. Chiropractic addresses the cause of interference in transmission of innate impulses. The chiropractic objective is to locate, analyze and facilitate the correction of vertebral subluxations for an innate-normal TRANSMISSION of innate impulses. The aim of the chiropractic objective is to restore the momentum of the transmission of innate impulses back to innate-normal. Nothing more. Nothing less. Nothing else. The living body is the greatest and most sophisticated device that we use on a daily basis to move, relate, and communicate with the world.

ART. 218. ASSURANCE OF PRACTICING THE CHIROPRACTIC OBJECTIVE

The instructions of the 33 principles of chiropractic's basic science and its conclusive objective describe, exactly and completely what chiropractic is, what chiropractic does, how and why chiropractic does what it does. Study the 33 principles. Reflect. Deeply think them through in order to become aware of what they really are. Experience their ability to give you freedom from preconceived ideas and notions of life.

We are, all of us, without condemnation, called to wake up to the absolute veracity of the 33 principles of chiropractic's basic science, because the 33 are the ultimate instructions that will guide our course to practice exclusively the chiropractic objective. Doing so, will lead to a greater awareness of our mission as chiropractors and will continuously keep our vision sharp and keen.

ART. 219. HOW TO BECOME AWARE

What is awareness? It is a process of the educated brain where the educated control (also called educated mind), which is the activity of the innate law in the educate brain, avails itself of innate impulses to tincture them into educated impulses for voluntary functions, including memory and will, to compare percepts and educational impressions.

What does this mean in practical terms? It means to watch, to observe deeply as you study the 33 principles of chiropractic's basic science. Observe what is going on: the trees, the grass, the plants, the animals, your breath, your thoughts, your feelings, which is essentially some of the levels of complexity of E/matter moving in and around you. It is basically the chiropractic meaning of existence (Prin. 2). You observe it. You store these educational impressions in your memory. Then as you continue your study of chiropractic, you will break out of your pre-conceived ideas, notions and rigid patterns, that our education, thoughts, beliefs, and words have imposed us. Those are interferences in the flow of freedom that stems from the past. Hopefully we will see that chiropractic surpasses our previous understanding of life. It will help us move beyond what we've learned from those around us. The first step is to unlearn what we think we already know. This will hopefully remove obstacles to the flow of our understanding of life and help to develop reflective thinking. In order to achieve this, one must use the educated brain, more specifically an aspect of educated intelligence called the will, to relearn differently. Then one has to be willing to be open, not to find something to confirm what one already thinks, but a willingness to discover something new.

For example, I remember listening to a practice member many years ago say to me, "I wish I had met you a long time ago. I never understood chiropractic as you explained it. I am 32 years old, I have a college degree, and never learned about interference in the nerves before. This is something different, something completely new to me. You know what? I realize I was wrong all my adult life. I did not know any of this." He had tears running down his face. This is what awareness is all about.

ART. 220. AWARENESS OF NON-MATERIAL REALITIES

At this point, it is necessary to discuss some fundamental understanding of non-material realities. First of all, a universal principle of organization is intrinsic to all E/matter (Prin. 1). Without it, E/matter would not be maintained in existence. The universal principle of organization is a fundamental organizing principle, which is the principle of continual existence. The function of the universal principle of organization is to organize information/F (Prin. 8). This fundamental principle organizes unlimited information/F, maintaining all E/matter in existence. Therefore, living E/matter is maintained in existence by this fundamental universal principle of organization (Prin. 1). The body of a living thing is governed by an essential extension of the universal principle of organization called the innate law of living things, which maintains it alive (Prin. 20, 21) if it is possible to do so according to universal laws (Prin. 24). Its function is to adapt universal information/F, invest it with new character, and reorganize it into innate information/F (coding) for all the tissue cells (Prin. 23). The innate law of living things can adapt an unlimited supply of universal information/F. The innate law of living things is a part of the universal principle of organization, in so far as it is intrinsic to the existence of all living E/matter in the entire universe. The innate law of living things is also a part from the universal principle of organization, in so far as it is only localized within the body of living things. The innate law can also be called the law of adaptation of living E/mater, which is an essential extension of the universal principle of organization. Basically, the innate law is a localized aspect of the universal principle of organization, and as such, it is "under" the rule, of the initial universal principle. As an example, Newton's third law of equal and opposite reaction is "under" the rule of his second law of acceleration of the law of gravity.[51] The innate law, which is non-material and maintains the body alive within the limits of E/matter (Prin. 20, 21, 24), is an essential extended continuation of the universal principle of organization that is also non-material, maintaining all E/matter in existence (Prin.1). The universal principle of organization is everywhere in the universe and the innate law of living things is everywhere within all living E/matter in the universe. The universal principle of organization and the innate law of living things are non-material. They are really one and the same. The innate law is simply the universal principle

adapting more complex levels and states of E/matter. We arbitrarily differentiate them, as a universal principle of organization and the innate law of living things, for our own understanding. It is exactly the same way when we differentiate the law of universal gravitation and the law of geometry which are actually one and the same. "Einstein's general relativity is a mathematically beautiful application of geometric ideas to gravitational physics." [52] All innate information/F must first be coded and assembled before being conducted through the nerve system or radiated from within all tissue cells. The innate law of living things functions through an operating system within the body that is called the innate field, which is also non-discrete (non-material.) It is within the innate field that innate information/F is coded and assembled. The innate field is supplied innate impulses and innate rays directly from the innate law. "It is a vital spot and cannot be DIS-EASED (lack ease). Its existence is actual, but its location is theoretical".[53] It is located within the body of the living thing wherever the innate law acts. There is no transmission of innate impulses from the innate law to the innate field. There is no need as both are non-discrete concepts located simultaneously everywhere in the body. For this reason, it always contains 100% coded and assembled innate impulses.

Since living E/matter is continually supplied innate information/F computed by the innate law in order to keep it alive (Prin. 21), the innate field as an operating system, is used for coding and assembling innate information/F. Some of the innate information/F will emerge, as innate impulses, in the physical brain for centralization and transmission to effectuate coordination of action through the nerve system as conductor. Some will emerge as innate rays/waves from within all the cells of the body for controlling cellular components to effectuate metabolism. The innate field is non-discrete because it is the "vital spot" of codifying and assembly of innate information/F of the innate law, which is everywhere within the body. Therefore, the operating system of the innate law of living things is the innate field, and it is everywhere within the body.

At the precise moment of the coding of the innate information/F by the innate law into innate impulses or innate rays/waves, they are assembled within the innate field for conduction through the nerve system for coordination of actions (Prin. 32), or for radiation from within the tissue cell controlling its intracell particulates for metabolism for use in the body (Prin. 23). Chiropractic is only concerned with the

---

51. Densmore, Dana (ed.), "Selections from Newton's Principia" USA:GreenCat Books an imprint of Green Lion Press. (2004) p.31

52. Ashtekar, Berger, Isenberg, and MacCallum (eds.) "Gravity is Geometry, after all. General Relativity and Gravation: A Centennial Perspective." Cambridge: Cambridge University Press. (2015) p. 347 doi: 10.1017/CB09781139583961.010

53. Stephenson, R.W., "Chiropractic Text Book." (Vol XIV) Davenport, IA: The Palmer School of Chiropractic. (1948) p. 13

innate-normal transmission of innate impulses for coordination of activities, exclusively, through the practice of its objective.

Why, then, is the principle of continuous supply and computation so central to the progress of the understanding of chiropractic in general? Because it provides a particularly effective way to find errors in the explanations of chiropractic and correct them.

It was previously mentioned that the axiom, "We cannot give what we do not have" is a truism. It is largely dependent upon two counterfactual properties of information/F: the possibility to be re-organized and the possibility to be copied. Everything that the educated intelligence can construct is a copy of something that already exists and that can be re-organized at a different level for practical use.

For example, when dusk sets on the shores of Cape May on the tip of south west New Jersey, an incredible spectacle unfolds before our eyes. As the twilight gives way to night, lights and sounds fill the air. The spectacle gradually gets darker and darker, until the whole oceanic horizon and the sky become pitch black. We begin to observe lights from boats and further out, ships that move across the ocean, their light signals showing through the darkness. Small private aircrafts fly through the starry sky and do the same as they enter a predetermined pattern to begin their approach at the local airport where its beacon's green light flicks on and off, on and off, to guide them to a safe landing. We hear music come from the venues on the boardwalk inviting those interested in having a drink to relax in the warm breeze coming from the beach.

Each of those observed objects display different behaviors, yet they all have something in common. The music and the lights from the boats, the airplanes, and the airport are all capable of carrying information/force. They are all signals. Whether it be the vibration of molecules propagating sounds to one's ear or the electromagnetic field transmitting photons interacting with the innate field of one's eye, they are adapted and coded into sensory impulses transmitted to one's physical brain through afferent sensory nerves for decoding. The main reason why human beings can construct these systems of signal-communication is because they can only construct what can be copied. What get constructed is usually a mirror-copy of the human body and its functions.

It is extremely important to understand that for educated intelligence to tincture innate impulses into educated impulse and to construct signals that are meaningful for us to use, it must apply a principle that already exists, and copy a modification of its information/F to construct the codes necessary for a message (like the beacon flicking its green light on and off, on and off to signal to an aircraft a clear approach to landing).

This truism works in reverse as well to facilitate our explanations of certain aspects of the inner workings of the innate law, which is a 100%/perfect software that continuously adapts and processes the information/F within the living body as a universal computer, according to universal laws. When we attempt to describe with flow charts how the innate law interfaces with the body, all we have to do is observe what we construct and understand that this construction was possible due to the properties of copy-ability and reorganization of information/F and E/matter. Our construction is a reorganized copy of its existence in principles (Prin. 1, 20). We actually reorganize information/F and E/matter and invest them with neweducated configurations to construct new designs of say, architectures and technologies. The same applies as we use the principle of continuous supply and computation (Prin. 33) to illustrate, at least in principle, a few basic flowcharts (cycles).

The understanding of this truism is the fundamental basis to reposition the chiropractic profession through this textbook, and firmly stand it on the solid bedrock of the 33 principles of chiropractic's basic science. One hundred years ago our ancestors were not privileged to have today's knowledge. However, even with knowing less than today, D.D. Palmer, B.J. Palmer, and Ralph W. Stephenson were able to illustrate, at least in principle, a few basic cycles (flowcharts). As they observed, they realized that most of those principles are absolute, immutable and constant. They became aware of non-material realities and they were able to construct a working knowledge of those principles.

ART. 221. INTEGRATING THE MISSING LINK

The differentiation of chiropractic's basic science from chiropractic philosophy and from chiropractic art through the 33 principles reveals with clarity the three aspects of chiropractic. The integration of those aspects requires that there be a link uniting them. The function of information/F is to unite the immaterial organizing principle and the material E/matter (Prin. 9). This scientific deduction stems from the fundamental universal principle of organization, which continually organizes information/F that provides all E/matter with its properties and actions to maintain it in existence. This supply of properties and actions is the result of instructive information/F organized by this fundamental principle (Prin. 1, 8, 10, 13). Information/F is the interface that unites the immaterial with the material. Information/F is the instruction necessary to unite the non-physical and the physical. It is this crucial point that maintains the whole universe in existence. Without instructive information/F there would be no possibility that the immaterial and the material could be united. Chiropractic's basic science is based on what is possible according to universal laws (Prin. 24). This universal instructive information/F gives rise to the periodic table. It is important to understand that every bit of existence is directly dependent upon universal instructive information/F organized by a universal principle of organization to be continually maintained. The function of the instructive information provided by the 33 principles of chiropractic's basic science is the link that unites chiropractic philosophy and the art of chiropractic. The instructive information of the 33 principles of chiropractic's basic science become the, hard to vary, explanation of why to practice exclusively the chiropractic objective. The 33 principles are congruent through and through. The 33 principles are essentially the ***G***uiding ***P***rinciples ***S****teering* ***S***ystem (GPSS) for chiropractors to stay on course as they practice the chiropractic objective.

ART. 222. INTER-CONNECTIVITY AND INTEROPERABILITY

The function of the innate law is always normal (Prin. 27) and one of the resulting outputs of that function is coordination of action of all the parts of the body for mutual benefit (Prin. 23) according to universal laws (Prin. 24). In order to have coordination of action, there must be interconnectivity between information/F and all the parts of the body in order to manifest mutual benefit of the whole body. As the innate law adapts universal information/F and E/matter for coordination of action of all the parts of the body for mutual benefit (Prin. 23), the congruency of instructive information/F necessary to coordinate all the parts of the body needs organizational interoperability.

Let us use computer data processing to demonstrate the transmission of innate impulses within the nervous system. It will also evidence that the body is truly a universal computer governed by the innate law as normal and perfect software (Prin. 27, 33) even though the total human being is more than the components of computer software and hardware. The body is the integrated motion system within which we live our life. It is true that "we cannot give what we do not have." We cannot invent or construct anything that does not already exist in the universe because existence is complete (Prin. 5). It must have the property of copy-ability (ability of being copied). It works from above-down-inside-out.

The innate law of living things adapts universal information/F and E/matter for use in the body so that all parts will have coordinated action for mutual benefit (Prin. 23). The innate law governs the body by adapting, coding, and computing inputs of information/F for metabolic use and coordination of action of all the parts of the body. The parts of the body are a set of agents interacting within a finite (Prin. 24) process for mutual benefit. An action loop is one of the foundational elements for this coordination principle (Prin. 23, 32). The innate impulse as instruction of input is transmitted from the physical brain (CPU) through the conducting efferent nerves (transmitters), and returns as trophic impulse/signal which is impression of output through the afferent nerves (transmitters) back to the physical brain (CPU) for coordination of actions of the body parts (receptors.) It is a continuous action loop. Coordination tasks can be delegated by the innate control through computational processes to manage dependencies of flow and instruction sharing among activities.

From what have learned in the last few years from data processing is that "fields programmable gate arrays (cells, organs, systems, etc.) consist of a large number of logic block programs (innate information/F) that can be configured and reconfigured, individually, to do a wide range of tasks. One logic block may do arithmetic, another signals processing, and yet another look things up in a table. The computation of the whole is a function of how the individual parts are configured. Fields programmable gates arrays (cells, organs, systems, etc.) can be reprogrammed to the desired functionality requirements after manufacturing".[54]

We now know that the language of neurons and synapses are connected to bodily functions.[55] It appears that the innate law is akin to software (operating system, application programs, coders, device drivers, network interface, etc.). Neurons are akin to computer hardware (CPU, transmitters, hardware platform interface, modulators, processors, microprocessors, receptors, feedback loop, etc.), and bodily functions are akin to the actions that a computer performs (in-putting data, processing instructions, out-putting data, etc.). This means that the computation of data (information/F) unites the software (organizing principle) with the manifestation of data (E/matter) demonstrating the function of information/F (Prin. 10). If the heart is a biological pump and the nose is a biological filter, then the physical brain is a biological central processing unit and the nerves are a conductive transmission network system. The central nervous system is basically a sophisticated hardware system used to compute and transmit innate information/F, governed by the innate law, for coordination of actions of all the parts of the organism (Prin. 23, 32).

---

54. Field Programmable Gate Array (FPGA) xilinx.com/products/silicon-devices/fpga/what-is-an-fpga.html (Jan 2021)

55. The Synpase. Khanacademy.org/science/biology/human-biology/neuron-nervous-system/a/the-synapse (2021)

ART. 223. CHIROPRACTIC'S BASIC SCIENCE

To be accepted as a science, chiropractic must satisfy certain criteria:

1. A systematically organized body of knowledge: chiropractic is comprised of 33 principles concluding into an absolute irrefutable objective.

2. An experimental method: applying the principle of a vertebral adjustment (Prin. 31b) to practice the chiropractic objective through the location, analysis, and facilitation of the correction of vertebral subluxation.

3. Reproducibility: of the locating, analyzing and facilitating the correction of vertebral subluxations through pre and post checks (chiropractic objective).

4. Testable, verifiable, or falsifiable hypotheses through the chiropractic objective concluded from the 33 principles.

5. Specific predictions from chiropractic applied science to achieve the chiropractic objective. The application of the principles of chiropractic's basic science is for living things, more specifically the living vertebrate body (Prin. 31).

6. Natural things as cells, organs, functional systems, and living bodies that provide a sequence of representations, in which each transmission of conducted information/F for coordination of activities is under an innate control to demonstrate the absolute necessity of correcting interference to the momentum of transmission (Prin. 29, 31a, 31b, 32).

What is central to the progress of chiropractic is the testability of predictions because it provides an effective way to find errors and make appropriate corrections through analytical pre-check and post-check.

In the book *A New Look at Chiropractic's Basic Science*, those criteria were analyzed and it was concluded that chiropractic's basic science met all of the criteria. It was also clarified that energy and matter are comprised of the same subatomic particles (electrons, neutrons, and protons) with different configuration and velocities ($E=mc^2$), making them interchangeable.[56] This means that energy and matter are one and the same. Therefore, force in chiropractic, which is the second factor of the Triune of Existence (Prin. 4), cannot be energy since energy is the mass of matter at the square of the speed of light ($E=mc^2$). Energy and matter are interchangeable. Force, in chiropractic, is information. Information is non-discrete.

In some respects, information/F is an abstraction of a particular principle, be it of an organized interstellar galaxy, of an organized universal computer, or of an organized body of a living thing. Information/F is organized in symbols in the form of codes in order to communicate a message. The innate law of the human body has always controlled and organized information/F, for use in every cell of the body, through adaptation, computation, and encoding (Prin. 20, 23). From this encoding information/F, it constructs new cells through its own computational methods.

That is precisely what the 33 principles of chiropractic's basic science are all about. The 33 principles are congruent with all of the laws of conservation, and they explain some aspect of the laws of motion as consequences of a universal regularity in nature. The chiropractic objective concluded from those 33 principles is to locate, analyze and facilitate the correction of vertebral subluxation for an innate-normal transmission of conducted innate information/F of the body.

56. Lessard, Claude. "A New Look at Chiropractic's Basic Science." (2014) Self Published. p.59

As an analogy, a receptor (receiving tissue cell) receives a message from a CPU computer (brain cell) through a medium, which is a transmitter (nerve cell). This explains that the receptor, computer, and transmitter are physical systems. It is a triunity that is a physical representation of the ADIO viewpoint. However, note that the message is not physical. The message is information/F initially organized, encoded, and assembled, as instructions in the computer. At this moment it is propelled through the transmitter and decoded by the receptor. The overall process constitutes, to the observer, what is possible in terms of adaptation and computation; it also points to a possibility of interference of the transmitting nerve due to limitations of E/matter and time (Prin. 6, 24, 29). This interference would alter the momentum of transmission of the innate impulse, thus altering the timing of the encoded data necessary for normal transmission of the message, and violating the principle of coordination (Prin. 6, 28, 29, 31a, 31b, 32).

This is an explanation of chiropractic that is hard to vary. This explanation constructs a solid universal platform that is based on universal principles and demonstrates what is possible all of the time. It is an invitation for you, the student, to focus on this explanation until the BIG IDEA engages you to make a connection with a larger vision. Sit with it, and if need be, read it again and again and again, and think it through until you feel its impact, until you can see its larger implications for the world, for history and for you until this explanation is transformed from a belief to a working knowledge within you. Become aware of it. In due time, it will transcend your knowledge and become wisdom. B.J. Palmer wrote in *The Value of Chiropractic*,

"... Do not fight against receiving the very things you need most. When a new subject is presented for your consideration, study the thing presented, resolve it into knowledge, put it thru a process of analysis and allow time to put it thru a process, which will ripen the knowledge into wisdom, and you will gain many ideas of value. Don't pay so much attention to mere education, to what "the book" says. Be your own judge, put it to the inner test. Concentrate upon knowledge, and you will be overjoyed to find that when the time comes for you to leave the P. S. C. you will be wiser than when you came".[57]

ART. 224. EFFERENT NERVES

Efferent nerves are the conducting pathways of innate impulses for coordination of activities and educated impulses for voluntary actions, from physical brain (CPU) to body part (receptor). It is the route of nerve axons from processing physical brain-CPU to receiving body part-receptor. Efferent nerves, anatomically, are bundled neuronal axons, which lead out of the physical brain (CPU). They exit the cranium by various foramina. Most of the cranial nerves exit by small openings in the cranium. The spinal cord leaves the cranium through the foramen magnum. The efferent nerves have their neurons organized such that their axons extend from the nerve cell body, which is located inside the ventral horn of the spinal cord, extending toward the periphery, and they can be interfered by vertebral subluxations. Bundles of axons are enclosed within a sheath and form the nerve.

Philosophically, efferent nerves are the nerve-axons-transmitters of innate impulses from physical brain to body part for coordination of activities. There can be a single axon or a multitude of axons involved. Anatomically, the nerve divides and subdivides to supply the tissues of its environment for coordination of activities of body parts (*See Fig. 31*).

57. Palmer, B.J., "The Value of Chiropractic." (1915) Davenport, IA: The Palmer School of Chiropractic Fountain Head. (1997 Reprint) p. 19-20

ART. 225. AFFERENT NERVES

Afferent nerves are the conducting pathways of trophic impulse/signal-feedback for coordination of activities. They transmit trophic impulses/signals from the receiving body part (receptor) to processing physical brain (CPU.) Afferent nerves represent the route of nerve axons from receiving body part-receptor to physical brain-CPU.

Sensory nerves are the afferent nerves from the special sense organs. They carry universal information/F that has been detected by the sense organ (sensor/application) and has been adapted, processed, and coded into sensory impulses by the innate law within the innate field through the sensor. The sensory impulses are transmitted through the sensory nerve to the physical brain-CPU to be decoded by the innate law within the innate field of the physical brain.

In the 1920s the afferent nerve was theoretical in the normal complete cycle (flowchart). In the 2020s the afferent nerve is known to carry trophic impulses/signals as feedback for coordination of activities and is not subject to interference in transmission from vertebral subluxation. This is because the nerve cell body is located in the dorsal root of the spinal nerve outside the spinal cord (*See Fig. 31*). The afferent nerve is always from receptors or sensors toward CPU. Its route is from periphery to central.

REVIEW QUESTIONS FOR ARTICLES 216 - 225

1. Explain why chiropractic is always at cause.
2. Which principle confirms chiropractic being always at cause?
3. What is the mission of the chiropractic profession?
4. What is the vision of the chiropractor?
5. What is the chiropractic objective?
6. What is the purpose of chiropractic?
7. What is awareness?
8. What process is involved in moving from knowledge to wisdom, according to B.J. Palmer, D.C.?
9. Is the innate law of living things a part of the universal principle of organization or a part from the universal principle of organization?
10. Where is the location of the universal principle of organization?
11. Where is the location of the innate law of living things?
12. What is the interface that unites the non-physical with the physical?
13. What is the guiding principles system (GPS) of the chiropractor?
14. What is the basis of the "hard to vary" explanation of chiropractic?
15. What are the criteria that chiropractic must satisfy to be accepted as a science?
16. State the chiropractic objective.
17. Which principle is to be applied by the chiropractor to exclusively practice the chiropractic objective?
18. What is the differentiation between efferent and afferent nerves?
19. Are sensory nerves efferent or afferent?
20. Why is an efferent nerve subject to vertebral subluxations and an afferent nerve is not?

ART. 226. SENSORY NERVES

Sensory nerves are afferent nerves conducting sensory impulses that are coded by the innate law within the sense organ. These sensory impulses are transmitted to the physical brain via sensory nerves for processing by the innate control. Those sensory impulses then undergo conscious interpretation through the educated brain. Sensory impulses are the necessary innate information/F to be used by the educated intelligence to further adapt the body to the external environment. The dendrites of sensory nerves are constructed of neurons that are sensors of specific universal information/F of the electromagnetic field, interacting with the innate field of those specific neurons, just like data processing applications (apps). Most of the special sense organs have cranial nerves as their sensory nerves.

A study of these flowcharts (*See Fig. 14, 15*) will show that special sense organs are always periphery in the normal complete cycle. As sensors they interact with universal information/F from the environment. A multitude of cycles operate simultaneously in the living body.

The sensory impulses are adapted information/F by the innate law and coded within the innate field of the sense organ to be transmitted through afferent nerves going to the innate field and educated field of the physical brain. Sensory impulses are coded innate information/F that are also transmitted through afferent nerves that are going only to the innate field of the physical brain. Sensory impulses are different and distinct from trophic impulses/signals coded for coordination of activities feedback.

Sensory impulses are coded information/F by the innate law for educated purposes in order for the individual to adapt to their environment, even while they sleep. They are conducted through afferent sensory nerves from the special sense organs (sight, hearing, taste, smell and touch) to inform the educated part of the physical brain regarding the environment. Since sensory impulses have an educated function, they can be subjected to interference, while trophic impulses/signals for coordination of activities feedback cannot be subjected to interference (*See Fig. 31*). Feedback for coordination of activities must always be true feedback, whether positive or negative.

ART. 227. SPECIAL SENSE

Special sense is the action from the special sense organs (sensors) that provides environmental information/F, which are adapted and coded into sensory impulses by the innate law, within the eye, nose, tongue, ear and skin to be transmitted through afferent sensory nerves. Special sense (sensor) is a sensory function, one of the nine primary functions. The five special senses are sight, smell, taste, hearing, and feeling.

ART. 228. SENSE OF EQUILIBRIUM AND ORIENTATION

The sense of equilibrium is encoded information/F into sensory impulses from the innate law using sensors of the inner ear to give a sense of balance. Those sensors are comprised of stereocilia to sense head position, head movement and body movements.

The sense of orientation is encoded information/F into sensory impulses from the innate law using sensors of the inner ear. Those special senses are specific to the semicircular canals of the inner ear comprised of three rings of the vestibule for orientation. One ring is for the horizontal plane and the other two are for the vertical plane. These sensory impulses are transmitted through the cochlear nerve, which is an afferent pathway, to the brain stem and cerebellum to be decoded and processed by the innate law, in the appropriate part of the physical brain allowing educated perception of equilibrium.

ART. 229. GENERAL SENSE

General sense is information/F coded by the innate law within the cell itself, as trophic impulses/signals, to be transmitted through afferent nerves for feedback to the physical brain for coordination of activities of the parts of the body. The trophic impulse/signal feedback is dependent on the soundness of the tissues of the body part as well as the innate-normal transmission of innate impulses for coordination of activities. Trophic impulses/signals are innate information/F describing the complete state of metabolism of the tissues of the body part and whether or not it has coordination of activities. They are received over the afferent half of the normal complete cycle. This innate information/F comprises a full indication of the soundness of the tissue that emanates from its specific motion, moment by moment, which reveals its complete biological properties, body chemistry and physiological actions. Those indications are, at times, manifested educationally in terms of conscious hunger, thirst, comfort, satisfaction, pleasure, etc. They are known educationally through the inter-field cycle (*See Fig.15*).

Pain, itching, and the like are subjective educated information/F of abnormalities in the periphery, via the inter-field cycle and normal complete cycle. They are both physiological sensations and emotional reactions to those sensations. It is perceived as a threat to the integrity of bodily soundness or vitality. The main role of pain is to help us make educated choices regarding tissue damage through modified trophic impulses/signals coded by the innate law that includes specific aspect of the soundness of the tissues involved. These modified trophic impulses/signals are transmitted through the afferent nerves. They are decoded within the innate field of the physical brain and made known educationally through the educated brain.

ART. 230. ORGANIZATION

Organization is an assemblage of universal information/F providing properties and actions to an entity, such as E/matter in order to maintain it in existence (Prin. 1). The human body is a superb organization with definite centralization at the physical brain for coordination of activities of all its parts for mutual benefit (Prin. 23). Each part has a role and a purpose to fulfill with coherent activities in order to satisfy the principle of coordination (Prin. 32) for use in the body by the innate law to maintain the body alive (Prin. 19, 21, 23).

The Merriam-Webster dictionary defines *organize* as:

> **1:** To form into a coherent unity or functioning whole: INTEGRATE
>
> **2a:** to set up an administrative structure
>
> **b:** to persuade to associate in an organization
>
> **3:** to arrange by systematic planning and united effort
>
> **4:** to cause to develop an organic structure

From this definition, an organism is maintained in existence through its being organized (Prin. 1), which is the initial condition of chiropractic's basic science, namely, "A universal principle of organization is continually supplying properties and actions to all E/matter, thus maintaining it in existence." As the states and levels of E/matter become more complex and move from condensed E/matter of non-living things to freely adaptable E/matter of living things, an essential extension of this universal principle of organization is the innate law of living things (Prin. 20).

Existence, being perfect (Prin. 5), is simply the expression of organization through E/matter (Prin. 2). It is E/matter that expresses the information/F of this principle of organization (Prin.13), which is then manifested through the motion of E/matter (Prin. 14). The innate law of the living body (Prin. 20) is perfect (Prin. 22). Its purpose is to maintain materials of the living body alive (Prin. 21) through adaptation (Prin. 23) only if it is possible according to universal laws (Prin. 24).

Previous volumes illustrated that organization bespeaks intelligence. What is the hard to vary explanation of chiropractic philosophy regarding the organizing principle? It is that the universal principle of organization is caused by intelligence, a universal intelligence. What is then the cause of this universal intelligence? This question is outside of the realm of chiropractic philosophy. It is in the realm of theology. Chiropractic is not theology. Chiropractic is a philosophy, a science, and an art.

REVIEW QUESTIONS FOR ARTICLES 226 - 230

1. What are sensory nerves?
2. Does the special sense cycle work while we sleep?
3. What is special sense?
4. What primary function is special sense?
5. Name the different kinds of feelings?
6. What is general sense?
7. Give an example of a normal general sense?
8. Give an example of an abnormal general sense?
9. Why are we educationally conscious of abnormal general senses sometimes?
10. What is the difference between general sense and special sense?
11. What does the term organize signifies?
12. What is the universal principle of organization?
13. What is the innate law of living things?
14. Is chiropractic a theological construct?

ART. 231. COORDINATION

Coordination is the perfect coherence of actions of all the parts of an organism for mutual benefits. It is the result of all the computations of the innate law governing the instructive information of innate impulses and the momentum of the flow of the transmission of innate impulses. Innate computation of universal information/F is an adaptation encoding an infinite number of innate impulses as input instructions for coordination of action of all the parts of the body as manifested output. It is about coherence, meaning a consistent balance of actions. Otherwise, if the momentum of the innate impulses is interfered by vertebral subluxations, the instructive information/F of the innate impulse will be received at the receptor part "out of timing" (Prin. 6, 29, 31a). Then it will have a proportion of time quality which is nothing less than mere non-adapted universal information/F, unable to balance properly the information/F already in the tissues of the receptor part. This will cause in-coordination of action of the receptor part. This will bring about a lack of coherence of biological activities and, thus, violate the principle of coordination (Prin. 32).

It is the practice of the chiropractic objective to apply the principle of a vertebral adjustment (Prin. 31b) through a specific adjustic thrust to facilitate the correction of a vertebral subluxation. This will restore the momentum of transmission of innate impulses (Prin. 29), thus satisfying the principle of coordination (Prin. 32) and bring about coherent activities of all the parts of the living body (Prin. 23).

ART. 232. FUNCTION AND FUNCTIONING

According to the 33 principles of chiropractic's basic science, chiropractic only has one function in the body which is removing interference in transmission of innate impulses for coordination of activities, exclusively through the correction of vertebral subluxations (Prin. 29, 30, 31, 32). Once a vertebral subluxation is detected by the chiropractor, the sole objective is to analyze it in order to introduce a specific adjustic thrust for the facilitation of a vertebral adjustment by the innate law (Prin. 31a, 31b). Chiropractic does not concern itself with the functions of the body part-receptor (Prin. 33). Chiropractic restores the momentum of transmission of conducted information/F through the practice of its objective in order to satisfy the principle of coordination (Prin. 32).

Note to the student: The following articles (Art. 232 – Art. 244) are written for the student to gain a greater appreciation of chiropractic, inasmuch as chiropractic does not concern itself with the actual function of the body parts except that their innate impulses are received without interference by vertebral subluxation for coordination of activities. It also reinforces the necessity for chiropractors to practice the chiropractic objective exclusively.

Function is the action of any existing thing in the universe. It is the purpose for which a thing exists. Functioning is the actualization of that purpose.

The Merriam-Webster dictionary defines *function* as:

1: Professional or official position: occupation

2: The action for which a person or thing is specially fitted or used or for which a thing exists;

3: Any of a group of related actions contributing to a larger action especially: the normal and specific contribution of a bodily part to the economy of a living organism

The manner in which a living thing functions, relies upon the information it receives in order to be functioning according to universal laws. Living things have limitations. Every cell of every part within the living body has a function and is dependent upon the innate information/F it receives for adequate functioning. Basically, every tissue cell receives innate impulses for coordination of activities and innate rays/waves for its metabolism. Chiropractic's only concern is to remove interference to the momentum of the transmission of innate impulses, through the practice of its objective so that all the parts of the body will function with coordination of activities for mutual benefit (Prin. 6, 23, 29, 31a, 31b, 32). The function of the innate law is always normal as the innate law is always normal (Prin. 27). It is always 100%/perfect (Prin. 22) and as a principle it has no limitations and will adapt information/F and E/matter perfectly only if it is possible within the limitations of E/matter (Prin. 23, 24).

ART. 233. FUNCTION OF THE INNATE LAW OF LIVING THINGS

Function of the innate law, which is an essential extension of the universal principle of organization, is to adapt universal information/F and E/matter for use in the body (Prin. 23). The innate law assembles, adapts, and codes information/F into innate impulses and innate rays/waves for use in the body.

Everything in the universe has a function, including the innate law. The basis for the existence of this extension of the universal principle of organization, called the innate law of living things, is an assemblage of (bits) unit-particles of E/matter of ever more sophisticated complex properties and actions which demonstrate highly organized manifestations that give rise to the ability of E/matter to be adaptable. Continuous adaptation of the body of living things is the essential function of the innate law to maintain it in active organization, to maintain it alive according to universal laws (Prin. 21, 23, 24). Adaptation is one of the signs of life (Prin. 18). For E/matter to be living, it must be adapted (Prin. 20, 21, 23). Without being adaptable it remains non-living E/matter.

Volume 1 and 2 illustrate that organization of particles of E/matter living and non-living things bespeaks intelligence. The function of the universal principle of organization is to organize information/F to provide properties and actions to all the bits of E/matter in order to continually maintain them in existence (Prin. 8). The function of the innate law adapts some bits of E/matter to maintain it living for a lifetime (Prin. 21, 23). The function of an organizing principle is an intelligent function.

ART. 234. THE FUNCTION OF A BODY

The function of a body is to express the information/F of the organizing principle (Prin. 13) and manifest it as a living thing (Prin. 18, 20) to complete the design of existence (Prin. 14, 15).

Everything in the universe, including the human body, has a function. According to the principles of chiropractic's basic science, the fundamental function of the body is to satisfy the principle of coordination (Prin. 32) through its expression of innate information/F (Prin. 13). For that to occur, it must have an innate-normal momentum in transmission of innate impulses. This fundamental function underscores the importance for chiropractors to exclusively practice the chiropractic objective.

ART. 235. THE FUNCTION OF AN ORGAN

The function of an organ is to express innate information/F (Prin. 13) which is to be manifested through coherent organized actions for the mutual benefit of all the body parts, hence the term "organ" (Prin. 14, 23). The purpose of an organ is to satisfy the principle of coordination (Prin. 32). The function of any part of the body is to express innate information/F in order to manifest coordination of activities to benefit the organization of the whole body (Prin. 13, 14, 23, 32). An organ is a receptor part that is adapted and processed by the innate law to act in a coordinated manner to benefit the whole body. Chiropractic is not concerned with the metabolic condition of the organ-receptor. The practice of chiropractic is exclusively concerned with removing any interference in the momentum of transmission of innate impulses through the correction of vertebral subluxations (Prin. 31a, 31b). Doing so restores the transmission of conducted information/F back to innate-normal (Prin. 27) and satisfies the principle of coordination (Prin. 32).

REVIEW QUESTIONS FOR ARTICLES 231 - 235

1. What is coordination?
2. What is coordination in the body?
3. State principle 32.
4. What is function?
5. What is functioning?
6. Does chiropractic concern itself with function of the body per se?
7. What is the concern of chiropractic that interferes with function in the body?
8. What is the innate law's function in the body?
9. What is the basis for the existence of the innate law?
10. When does the innate law adapt the material of the body?
11. Why does the innate law adapt the material of the body?
12. Organization bespeaks what?
13. Is the function of an organizing principle an intelligent act?
14. What is the fundamental function of the body?
15. What is the function of an organ as a receptor?
16. What is it that benefits from the coordinated action of an organ?

ART. 236. THE FUNCTION OF A TISSUE CELL

A tissue cell is the smallest organized unit in the body. Its function is to express innate information/F (Prin. 13) which is manifested through coherent actions for mutual benefit of the entire body part which, in turn, benefits the organization of the whole body (Prin. 14, 23, 32).

The cell is the smallest definite unit of the body. It is within itself, a definite entity like the whole body itself. The intra-cell particulates (nucleus, mitochondria, lysosomes, ribosomes, golgi apparatus, etc...) are the cell's parts functioning for its own benefit. The intra-cell particulates are under the innate control through innate rays/waves and the body chemistry of the serous circulation. These functions of the intra-cell particulates are not functions of the whole body directly, but are functions of the tissue cell's body under direct control of the innate law intrinsic within the innate field of the cell itself. The manifestations of the functions of the intra-cell particulates are signs of life (Prin. 18). A single cell in a petri-dish can be kept alive for laboratory study or a heart can be kept alive in a chemical solution for transport in the case of a transplant. The functions of the intra-cell particulates benefit the whole body.

The cell is a sophisticated, specialized receptor to be processed by the innate law as 100%/perfect software for a specific computed type of work. The cell's structure and location are always according to the type of functional output that it is constructed to manifest. Each tissue cell may be used for several different kinds of output depending upon the computations necessary on a moment by moment basis to maintain the body alive in a state of coherent actions according to universal laws (Prin. 21, 24, 32).

Universal information/F of tissue cells manifest motion for dynamic purposes. To become functional and express its physiological purpose in the living body, a tissue cell must be adapted, computed, and coded into innate rays/waves (metabolism) and innate impulses (coordination of activities) by the innate law. We must remember that adaptability of cells in the body is a sign of life (Prin. 18) and, as such, adaptability is dependent upon the function of the innate law within the limitation of E/matter (Prin. 23, 24).

To be maintained in existence, a tissue cell expresses universal information/F that is manifested as universal motion (Prin. 1, 13, 14). For a tissue cell to be maintained alive and actualize its purpose, universal information/F must be adapted, computed and coded into innate information/F by the innate law (Prin. 20, 21, 23). When adapted, a tissue cell manifests a unique motion that is its functional purpose (Prin. 14). If it is not adapted, it acts without innate control and will not manifest its functional purpose. The cell will die and manifest only universal motion. This means that a tissue cell, living or non-living (necrosis), will always express universal information/F, through the configuration of its electrons, protons and neutrons that are continually maintained in existence (Prin. 1).

ART. 237. THE FUNCTION OF EPITHELIAL TISSUE

The function of epithelial tissue is dependent upon its specific purpose in the body. Its structural variations are according to the kind of outputs from their processed computations (secretory, protective, lining, conveying, etc.) The function of epithelial tissue may be active or passive.

Universal information/F of epithelial cells manifest motion for dynamic purposes. To become functional and express their physiological purposes in the living body, epithelial cells must be adapted, computed, and coded into innate rays/waves (metabolism) and innate impulses (coordination of activities) by the innate law.

ART. 238. THE FUNCTION OF CONNECTIVE TISSUE

The function of connective tissue is dependent upon its specific purpose in the body. Its structural variations are according to the kind of outputs from their processed computations (connecting, strength, support, etc.). The function of connective tissue is mainly passive. As part of active organs or glands it has active functions indirectly. Active or passive, its function is to benefit the whole organization of the living body through its participation in the coherence of all the parts of the body (Prin. 32).

Intra-cell particulates of each individual cell of connective tissues are under innate control for metabolism and vitality through innate rays/waves, including the body chemistry of the serous circulation. Each cell possesses the property of adaptability in order to be computed by the innate law which is a perfect innate software that is continuously supplied universal information/F from the universal principle of organization (Prin. 1, 33). Chiropractic does not address innate rays/waves, nor the body chemistry of the serous circulation. Chiropractic addresses exclusively interference in the momentum of transmission of innate impulses for coordination of activities (Prin. 28, 29, 30, 31a, 31b, 32).

ART. 239. THE FUNCTION OF MUSCLE TISSUE.

The function of muscle tissue is physiologic automation. Its purpose is to move the whole body or some its part for specific motion and as such it is always active. Every cell possesses the property of adaptability in order to be computed by the innate law which is a perfect innate software that is supplied continuous universal information/F from the universal principle of organization (Prin. 1, 20, 33). Through educated intelligence, an individual can tincture innate impulses and modify them into educated impulses for voluntary actions. This educated act is usually performed for the individual's adaptation to life circumstances both external and internal.

ART. 240. THE FUNCTION OF NERVE TISSUE

The function of nerve tissue is to conduct innate information/F. Some innate information/F are innate impulses for coordination of activities. Some information/F are trophic impulses/signals for motion of feedback of metabolism, soundness and activities. Some innate information/F are sensory impulses for educated adaption to the external environment. Some innate information/F are tinctured and modified into educated impulses for voluntary actions.

The law of continuous supply and computation is an inexhaustible source of universal information/F from which to code inforuns. Each cell possesses the property of adaptability in order to be computed by the innate law which is a perfect innate software that is supplied continuous universal information/F from the universal principle of organization (Prin. 1, 33). Chiropractic does not address innate rays/ waves. Chiropractic addresses exclusively interference in transmission of momentum of innate impulses for coordination of activities.

REVIEW QUESTIONS FOR ARTICLES 236 – 240

1. What is the function of a tissue cell according to the principles of chiropractic's basic science?
2. Is a tissue cell an entity?
3. Name some of the functions of epithelium.
4. Name the main function of connective tissue.
5. What other specific functions may connective tissue have?
6. What is the function of muscle tissue?
7. What other specific functions may muscle tissue have?
8. What is the main function of nerve tissue?
9. What other specific functions may nerve have?
10. What is the property that a cell must possess to be computed by the innate law?
11. Must the intra-cell particulates have coherence of actions within the cell?
12. What controls the coherence of actions of the intra-cell particulates?
13. What is the information/F coded by the innate law within the cell called?
14. What is the information/F coded by the innate law from the environment called?
15. What is the information/F tinctured by educated intelligence for voluntary actions called?
16. What is the kind of innate information/F that chiropractic exclusively deals with?
17. Why is it important to study functions of organs and glands of the body?

ART. 241. UNIVERSAL FUNCTION IN THE BODY

Universal function in the body is a universal law. It is organized universal information/F manifesting the motion involved in the configurations and velocities of electrons, protons and neutrons, which are the properties and actions of E/matter that is maintained in existence by the universal principle of organization (Prin. 1, 14). An essential extension of the universal principle of organization is the innate law of living things, the function of which is to adapt, code and compute universal information/F and E/matter for the mutual benefit of all the body parts, only if it is possible according to universal laws for a life time (Prin. 22, 23, 24). The innate control will not break a universal law.

When universal information/F is adapted by the innate law it becomes innate information/F, processed and coded, for maintaining the body alive within the limits of its adaptation (Prin. 22, 23, 24). If universal information/F is not adapted, it is deconstructive toward structural E/matter that it is a part of and breaks it down to its smallest component, which is the atom (Prin. 11, 26). Universal function is the manifestation of the universal principle of organization (Prin. 1, 14). It stems from the expression of organized universal information/F, which are the configurations and velocities of the electrons, protons and neutrons of the atoms manifested as motion (Prin. 1, 13, 14). The innate control adapts, computes, processes, and codes universal information/F into innate information/F for constructive use in the body to maintain it alive according to universal laws (Prin. 22, 23, 24).

ART. 242. GENERAL OR METABOLIC FUNCTION IN THE BODY

General or metabolic functions are manifestations of instructive information/F expressed by living E/matter to keep the tissue cell of the body alive in fulfilling its designed purpose according to universal laws (Prin. 13, 14, 21, 23, 24). The intra-cell particulates contained within the protoplasm of all living cells are in constant motion (Prin. 14, 15, 21). This is the expression of innate information/F that maintains the living cells alive as signs of life (Prin. 18) through innate rays/waves. This is what makes living E/matter distinct from non-living E/matter. The manifestations of the unique functions of all living cells stem from their expressions of universal information/F some of which have been adapted, computed and coded by the innate law into specific instructions to fulfill their definite purpose. There is within the body an equivalence of balance of both universal and innate information/F under the innate control. That is why metabolic functions are general functions in so far as they generally maintain each individual cell alive within their material limitations through innate rays/waves that provide the soundness and vitality of the cell. Chiropractic does not concern itself with innate rays/waves. These functions benefit the cell first then the body second. It is possible for a cell to be alive and not benefit the whole body, as in a cancer cell for example. For a cell to benefit the whole body, its functions must have coordinative actions, which result from an innate-normal flow of innate impulses through efferent nerves and its feedback flow of trophic impulses/signals through afferent nerves (*See Fig. 5*). Chiropractic concerns itself exclusively with the innate-normal momentum of transmission of innate impulses through the practice of its objective.

ART. 243. PRIMARY OR COORDINATIVE FUNCTIONS IN THE BODY

Primary or coordinative functions are manifestations of instructive information/F expressed by living E/matter for coordination of action of all the parts of the body for mutual benefit according to universal laws (Prin. 23, 24). Coordinative functions benefit the whole body in fulfilling their designed purpose if it is possible within the limits of the body's adaptability.

Since the tissue cell is the smallest unit of the body, it is the basic bit of biology in the study of function. In this sense, we study the meaning of function to help us grasp how amazingly mind boggling, and immensely breathtaking, is the multitude of flowcharts of adaptability that are continually computed and processed simultaneously, by the instantaneous integral innate adaptation, every factorial moment, according to universal laws. When all the parts of the body act coordinately, they manifest coherent actions through expressing innate information/F that have been received in a timely manner (Prin. 6, 23, 32).

Coordinative function of living E/matter manifests motion for coordination of activities of all the parts of the body, whereas metabolic function manifests motion for the soundness and vitality of the parts. Both are under absolute control of the innate law, and both are necessary to satisfy the principle of coordination (Prin. 32) in order to benefit the whole body (Prin. 23).

ART. 244. COORDINATIVE FUNCTIONS AND THEIR FEEDBACK

Coordinative functions have been arbitrarily divided into eleven kinds, for convenience, by R.W. Stephenson. The coordinative functions are general function, motor function, caloric function, sensory function, secretory function, excretory function, nutritive function, cellular replacement function, expansive function, reproductive function, transmission function, and connectivity function. Each function is generated from the expression of innate impulses that have been transmitted from the physical brain through efferent nerves that are received by the body parts (receptors) and have been manifested by specific motions. These functional motions are then coded into trophic impulses/signals through afferent nerves for feedback to the physical brain (CPU). Feedback is necessary for coordination of activities of all the body parts for mutual benefit. Both efferent and afferent paths of the normal complete cycle (flowchart) are vital to satisfy the principle of coordination (Prin. 32). Most of the coordinative functions are the collaborative actions of many tissues as they are manifestations of the expression of innate information/F from living E/matter for coordination of activities continuously adapted by the innate law within the limitation of E/matter (Prin. 23, 32). Chiropractic does not address functions of body parts. Chiropractic addresses only the restoration of transmission of innate impulses through the practice of its objective (Prin. 29, 30, 31a, 31b).

ART. 245. THE PRINCIPLE OF CONTINUOUS SUPPLY AND COMPUTATION

All tissue cells of the living body are continuously supplied information/F since they are continually maintained in existence (Prin. 1). When a tissue cell has the property of adaptability it will be continually adapted, computed, and processed by innate control for mutual benefit of all body parts for coordination of activities according to universal laws (Prin. 23, 24). The motions manifested by the tissue cell are coded into trophic impulses/signals for feedback that includes the quality of the soundness of the tissue cell and the state of its coordinative actions. Those trophic impulses/signals are impressions of vibrations containing information/F (universal and innate) about the soundness of the cell and its activities. The afferent nerve, which is not subject to vertebral subluxations, transmits the trophic impulses/signals waving instructive signals through the innate field to the physical brain. There, they are decoded by the innate control in order to construct, within the innate field, the vital innate impulses, the vital innate rays/waves, producing the vital body chemistry through the serous circulation, from all the appropriate tissue cells of the body, thus computing and processing the feedback. It is understood that body chemistry through the serous stream requires more time to be supplied (Prin. 6). This is a continuous supply and computation for the entire lifetime of each cell the body within its limits of adaptability (Prin. 6, 23, 24). Universal information/F is continuously supplied to the body (as a living computer) and every one of its parts (as receptors). Each body part is continuously adapted and computed by the 100%/perfect innate law (100%/perfect software) through the innate field (operating system) using the physical brain (CPU) and brain cells (processors) to code information/F into innate impulses (message) to be transmitted through the nerves (transmitters) for coordination of activities.

It is the coded trophic impulses/signals by the innate law that is the feedback for centralization and processing in the physical brain for coordination of activities. It is always the 100%/perfect innate control that governs the activities of body parts, including the tinctured innate impulses into educated impulses for voluntary actions, according to universal laws (Prin. 20, 23, 24, 32). It underscores the importance of practicing exclusively the chiropractic objective, which is the location, analysis and facilitation of the correction of vertebral subluxations for an innate-normal transmission of innate impulses.

REVIEW QUESTIONS FOR ARTICLES 241 - 245

1. What is universal function?
2. What is the characteristic of universal function outside the body?
3. What does the innate law do with universal information/F in the body?
4. What happens if universal information/F is not adapted in the body?
5. What is metabolic function in the body?
6. What is the difference between metabolic function and universal function?
7. What is coordinative function in the body?
8. What is the difference between metabolic function and coordinative function?
9. Name the kinds of arbitrary coordinative functions in the body.
10. Why do chiropractic students study the meaning of function in the body?
11. State principle 33.
12. Explain the work of principle 33.
13. Why is there a continuous supply of universal information/F in the body?
14. What is the coded feedback of body part activities called?
15. Through which nerves are trophic impulses/signals transmitted?
16. Are afferent nerves for coordination of activities subject to vertebral subluxation? Why?
17. What manifested output product requires more time to be supplied as input to the cell for metabolism?

ART. 246. NORMAL FUNCTION

The only normal function in the body of living things is called innate-normal. Only the innate law, which is an extension of the universal principle of organization (Prin. 1, 20), is normal and its function is always normal (Prin. 27). The function of the universal principle of organization and its essential extension, the innate law, are always 100%/perfect (Prin. 5, 22). On the other hand, all the tissue cells of the parts of the body are subject to the limitation E/matter (Prin. 24). There is always imperfection of the E/matter in the body of living things. Therefore, perfection of body functions is not possible due to the limits of adaptability of living E/matter. The best that chiropractic can do is to restore the transmission of innate impulses through the practice of its objective. Chiropractic is always about what is possible, which is its objective. For example, a person in subzero temperature would not survive very long in shorts and T-shirt. The polar bear will survive in that environment without shorts and T-shirt. The innate law will always perfectly adapt living E/matter, moment by moment, according universal laws (Prin. 22, 23, 24).

The principle of continuous supply and computation is intrinsic to the body of living things (Prin. 33). It causes living E/matter to be continuously adaptable by the innate law, which is an extension of the universal principle of organization (Prin. 20, 23). The innate law is limited by the limitations of E/matter (Prin. 24). Interference in transmission of innate impulses due to vertebral subluxations further limits living E/matter and will cause it to be less adaptable. Within the triune, the interference in transmission of innate impulses is always between E/matter and E/matter, between the physical brain and the physical body part. The interference is never between the innate law and E/matter (Prin. 4, 29). The interference is WITHIN information/F, the second factor of the triune. The interference is the altered momentum of transmission of innate impulses. A vertebral subluxation causes a lack of ease of the transmitting neurons and the momentum of the transmission of innate impulses is altered. This interference in turn causes an untimely reception of the innate impulses at the receptor body part, thus compromising through an untimely reception of the instructive information/F that it carries (Prin. 6, 28, 29 30, 31a). The principle of coordination is thus violated (Prin. 32). Chiropractic is about satisfying the principle of coordination (Prin. 32) through the correction of vertebral subluxations (Prin. 31a, 31b) for the restoration of the transmission of innate impulses back to innate-normal (Prin. 27). This underscores the importance for chiropractors to practice the chiropractic objective exclusively.

When we observe that adaptation of living E/matter occurs moment by moment, it means that the innate law has always 100%/perfect function to continuously govern living E/matter, which is always imperfect, according to universal laws (Prin. 22, 23, 24, 33). The innate law is always normal and its function is always normal (Prin. 27).

A body part may act and does act under stimuli, but stimuli are not innate impulses and the action they cause is not coordinative for the benefit of the whole body. Only actions of body parts under innate control can be coordinated for mutual benefit (Prin. 23). Whether the function of a body part is innate-normal is totally dependent upon innate control. Educated intelligence is absolutely clueless regarding innate-normal function of body parts. All one can do with certainty for the body to have innate-normal functions, moment by moment, is to restore transmission of innate impulses through the location, analysis, and facilitation of the correction of vertebral subluxations, which is the chiropractic objective. Innate-normal body functions are the right functions for the internal and external circumstances of the moment that must be computed and processed according to universal laws. Circumstances continuously change. The functions of the body parts continuously vary as well and they are adapted by the innate law, through its 100%/perfect instantaneous integral adaptation. The innate law governs every function of the body (Prin. 23). The law of continuous supply and computation causes the continued possibility of adaptability of living E/matter to be adapted, computed, processed, and coded by the innate control, as 100%/perfect software according to universal laws (Prin. 23, 24, 33). Besides this, the body part must be sound and vital in order to function according to the instructive information/F of the innate impulse since the innate law is limited by the limitations of E/matter (Prin. 24). It is the limitation of E/matter and time, the lack of soundness, and the interference in transmission of innate impulses for coordination of activities that will prevent the tissue cells of the body part to function innate-normal.

It underscores the immense responsibility of the chiropractor to exclusively practice the chiropractic objective, which is based on the 33 principles of chiropractic's basic science.

Since it is only the function of the innate law of living things that is normal in the body, it is now necessary for the student to study the function of this innate law as an essential extension of the universal principle of organization, which is the initial condition of chiropractic's basic science.

Volumes 1 and 2 mentioned that organization bespeaks intelligence. Therefore, the fundamental cause of the universal principle of organization is a universal intelligence. Rational logic and deductive reasoning assert that the innate law of living things is also caused by a universal intelligence. This universal intelligence is separate and distinct from its universal principle of organization, which includes the innate law of living things. It is like the software engineer whose job is to design the software that will operate a computer. The engineer is separate from the computer and the software that runs it. Most users do not know the software engineer, yet they routinely utilize their devices.

The universal principle of organization is a scientific principle, the function of which is to organize information/F that supplies properties and actions to all E/matter, through the continual organization of its electrons, protons, and neutrons, in order to maintain it in existence (Prin. 1). Chiropractic appropriates this universal principle of organization as its major premise (Prin. 1). As more complex levels of organization evolve, we encounter living E/matter. As an essential extension of the universal principle of organization is the innate law of living things, the purpose of which is to maintain the material of the body of a living thing alive (Prin. 21). The innate law fulfills its purpose through its function, which is to adapt information/F and E/matter for use in the living body, so that all parts of the body will have coordinated actions for mutual benefit according to universal laws (Prin. 23, 24).

ART. 247. THE INNATE LAW AS A PRINCIPLE OF ADAPTATION (FUNCTION)

Universal information/F is continuously supplied to E/matter to maintain it in existence (Prin. 1). For condensed non-living E/matter, the computation of properties and actions is straightforward. It is the configuration of electrons, protons, and neutrons including their velocities that maintains E/matter in existence. For more complex living E/matter, the computation involves adaptation of universal information/F and E/matter to be maintained alive, for a lifetime, according to universal laws (Prin. 21, 23, 24). Living E/matter is also continuously undergoing computation to be maintained in continuous existence at the molecular level by the universal organizing principle.

One of the major areas of the development of chiropractic philosophy resides in the application of the information/F paradigm. You have encountered this paradigm previously when we demonstrated that force, in chiropractic's basic science, is information. This was concluded from the famous equation of Einstein, $E = mc^2$, where energy and matter are an interchangeable equivalence. Thus, the chiropractic lexicon includes the terms "information/F" and "E/matter."

Information/F is continually organized into instructions by the organizing principle. Specialized coding language of these instructions organize more and more complex properties and actions that give rise to living structures of E/matter with the property of adaptability, which is a sign of life (Prin. 18).

Through its normal function of adaptation, the innate law computes and processes universal information/F, transforming it into innate information/F. Innate information/F is coded into instructive innate rays/waves for metabolism, or innate impulses and innate trophic impulses/signals for coordination of activities, or innate sensory impulses for environmental adaptation, or innate impulses that have been tinctured into educated impulses for voluntary action. It is through these instructive innate information/F that the innate law governs living E/matter. All nine primary functions and all other functions are all directly governed by innate control for the benefit of the whole body. Therefore, there is absolutely no need for chiropractors to address any of these functions. For this reason, chiropractic addresses only interference in the momentum of the transmission of the innate impulses through the practice of its objective so that all the bodily functions will have innate-normal adaptation.

ART. 248. THE INFORMATION PARADIGM (INNATE ADAPTATION)

Chiropractic has paved the way through apprehending the innate law of living things with its firm instructions to E/matter for its practical starting point. In doing so, chiropractic aims to continually gain progressive working knowledge features of the interference to the transmission of innate impulse-messages (Prin. 20, 29). At this more complex level of organization of living E/matter, there exists a distinct demarcation between chiropractic philosophy and chiropractic science that is complementary. Chiropractic's basic science is useful to chiropractic philosophy and chiropractic philosophy is useful to chiropractic's basic science. Chiropractic's basic science starts with the fundamental universal principle of organization that maintains all non-living and living E/matter in existence (Prin. 1). D.D. Palmer wrote, "Chiropractic is the name of a classified, indexed knowledge of successive sense impressions of biology, the science of life, which science I created out of principles which have existed as long as vertebrate".[58] In practice however, chiropractic philosophy starts with the innate law of living things that maintains only living E/matter alive (Prin. 20, 21). This is derived from the founder of chiropractic, D.D. Palmer, who wrote that chiropractic is about the living body, "... to replace displaced vertebrae by using the spinous and transverse processes".[59] Therefore, the initial principle of chiropractic philosophy in practice is the innate law of living things (Prin. 20). The previous 19 principles are fundamentals of existence. Chiropractic philosophy was developed through insights regarding the innate law of living things generated by information interactions. Through the appropriate steps of these interactions (processing, coding, assembly and dissemination of innate information/F), it became progressively what we call chiropractic philosophy in practice involving living E/matter through adaptation events based on well-defined interaction patterns. This venture involved the investigation and development of more or less insightful understanding of the organizing principle capable of adapting specific universal information/F and E/matter with perfect efficiency and computation.

Article 220 demonstrates examples of carriers of information (beacon light, music sound, food odor, etc.). They are all signals. They can carry information. This property possesses a unique class of systems in our universe called information media. Information is non-discrete, which means that it is not physical. Information is a code to be interpreted. For example, green light means go, red light means

58. Palmer, D.D., "The Chiropractic Adjuster. The Science, Art, and Philosophy of Chiropractic." Portland, OR: Portland Printing House. (1910) p. 1

59. Palmer, D.D., "The Chiropractic Adjuster. The Science, Art, and Philosophy of Chiropractic." Portland, OR: Portland Printing House. (1910) p. 280

stop. Any color of the spectrum emits photons of a particular frequency that strike your retina to be immediately adapted into innate sensory impulses to be conducted by the afferent optic nerve to the optic center of the physical brain for interpretation. When the interpretation is "green" the information code is "go." The photons and frequency, the retina sensor, the optic nerve conductor, the physical brain interpreter, they are all physical. But, the interpretation of the code is not physical. It is an assignment of an "agreed upon" coded message, in this instance "go." It could be anything you assign to it. It is merely an educated determination. Furthermore, this non-discrete information can be copied. Everyone can duplicate the information of the color "green" as meaning "go." Since information can be carried and copied by a physical system (you), the information acquires a physical reality. This literally means that the information/F being conducted by the nerve system becomes both non-discrete (innate) and discrete (impulse). It is a non-physical message being carried through a physical medium.

ART. 249. INNATE IMPULSE (INNATE ADAPTATION)

Innate impulse is both non-physical and physical whose origin is the innate field, which is non-local. The innate field is that non-discrete aspect of the body that is utilized by the innate law, as an operating system, to assemble, to adapt, to code, and to characterize universal information/F into innate information/F. The innate field is operated by the innate law to assemble innate information/F for use in the body and for coordination of activities (Prin. 23). It is supplied with innate information/F to function directly from the innate law. It is the operating system of the innate control to govern everything in the body. It is vital and cannot lack ease since it is 100%/perfect. It is non-discrete, as is the innate law and has no material component. This means that the innate field is a non-discrete, metaphysical construct. Its location is wherever the innate law is in the body, which is everywhere within the body. Its existence is actual, it is vital, and it is operated by the innate control. It has no material component. The innate field is a metaphysical construct. It is where the non-material instructive codes of the innate impulse originate. It is the interface where the metaphysical instructions of the innate information/force unite the non-material innate law with the material E/matter.

The physical manifestation of the innate impulse in the body occurs through its material conductor, which is comprised of nerve tissue. The innate impulses assembled in the innate field of the physical brain are conducted through the spinal cord and spinal nerves manifesting the physical aspect of the innate impulse. From the physical brain, the innate law utilizes efferent neurons for transmission of the innate impulse to the receptor body part for coordination of activities.

ART. 250. INNATE SENSORY IMPULSES (INNATE ADAPTATION)

A sensory impulse is discrete. It is a universal information/F. Its origin is the external environment. Immediately upon impacting the living body, the sensory impulse is adapted into an innate-sensory impulse by the innate law becoming both non-discrete and discrete. The origin of the innate-sensory impulse is in the innate field, which is non-local. Innate-sensory impulses are especially coded by the innate law in order to provide data and inform the educated brain of environmental conditions. This data is used by the educated intelligence of individuals to become aware of its external environment in order to effectively adapt to their circumstances.

REVIEW QUESTIONS FOR ARTICLES 246 - 250

1. What is the only normal function in the body?
2. Which specific principle of chiropractic's basic science stipulates this fact?
3. Is the action caused by a stimulus coordinative? Why or why not?
4. Does "innate-normal" vary according to changes in circumstances?
5. Is living E/matter ever perfect in the body?
6. What is the fundamental cause of the universal principle of organization?
7. What does the computation of universal information/F of non-living E/matter entails?
8. What further step is computing universal information /F of living E/matter?
9. What is force in chiropractic?
10. What do beacon lights, aircrafts lights, music sounds, food odors, and innate impulses have in common?
11. Name the types of adapted universal information/F coded into innate information/F.
12. What is the purpose of innate impulses?
13. What is the purpose of innate rays/waves?
14. What is the purpose of innate trophic impulses/signals?
15. Chiropractic addresses exclusively which type of innate information/F? Why?
16. Is information discrete or non-discrete?
17. When does the innate impulse become both non-discrete and discrete?
18. What are the two properties that allow the innate impulse to be both?
19. Is the innate field local or non-local?
20. Why is the innate field a metaphysical construct?
21. Is a sensory impulse discrete or non-discrete?
22. Is an innate-sensory impulse discrete or non-discrete?
23. When does a sensory impulse become an innate-sensory impulse?
24. What is the purpose of innate sensory-impulses?

ART. 251. INTER-CONNECTIVITY AND INTEROPERABILITY (INNATE ADAPTATION)

The innate law of living things adapts universal information/F and E/matter for use in the body so that all parts will have coordinated action for mutual benefit (Prin. 23). The innate law governs the body by adapting, computing, and coding inputs of information/F for metabolic use and coordination of action of all the parts of the body. The parts of the body are a set of agents interacting within a finite biological system (Prin. 24) for mutual benefit. An action loop is one of the foundational elements for this coordination principle (Prin. 23, 32). Based on the fact that, "we can only construct that which exists and can be copied in principle," this is what the theory proposes: Innate impulses, as input, are transmitted from the physical brain (CPU) through the conducting efferent nerves (neuron-transmitters located inside the ventral horn of the spinal cord), and return as trophic impulses/signals, which are impressions (feedback), as output, through the afferent nerve to the neuron-transmitter cell body located outside the spinal cord. From the afferent nerve cell body, the trophic impulse/signal then waves its way through the innate field back to the physical brain (CPU) for coordination of actions of the body parts (receptors). It is an action loop. Coordination relies include the soundness of the tissue cells of the body parts through innate rays/waves for metabolism and can be delegated through computational processes to manage dependencies of flow and instruction sharing among activities. Chiropractic addresses the transmission of innate impulses exclusively.

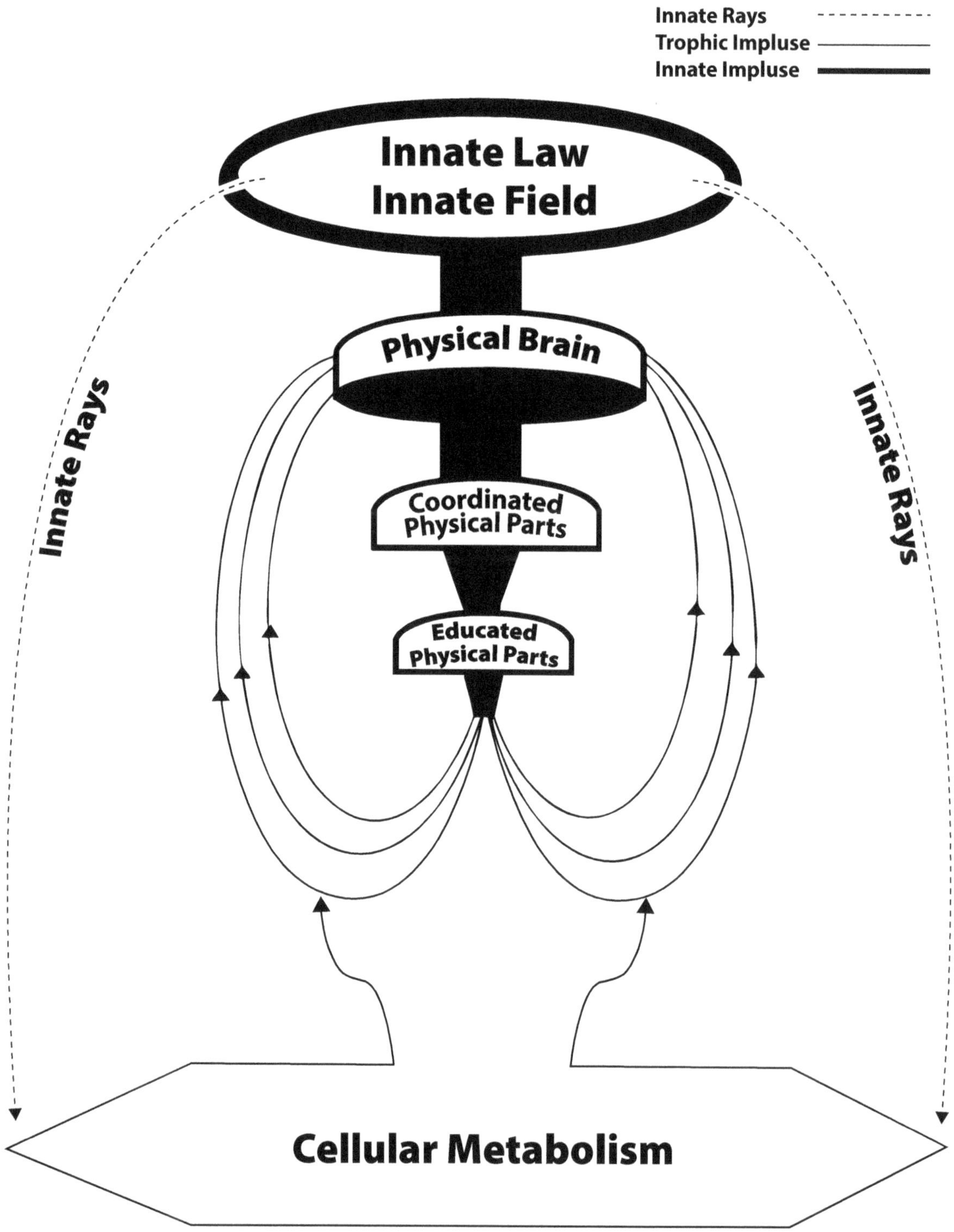

Fig. 32. Transmission of innate impulses through nerve conduction from physical brain to physical parts for coordination of activities, and innate rays through radiation from within every tissue cell controlling cellular components for metabolism, including trophic impulses/signals feedback loop to the physical brain.

This demonstration of interoperability through interconnectivity of the innate law reveals a complex level of organization of living E/matter that is continuously adapted, for each moment. It includes adaptation of information/F and E/matter for use in the body and for coordination of action of all the parts of the body for mutual benefit (Prin. 23).

ART. 252. COMPUTATION ANALOGY OF INNATE ADAPTATION

From what scientists have learned in recent years from data processing, we know that, "fields programmable gate arrays (biologically it would be the innate field of cells, organs, systems, etc.) consist of a large number of logic block programs (biologically it would be: innate information/F) that can be configured and reconfigured individually, to do a wide range of tasks. One logic block may do arithmetic, another signals processing, and yet another look things up in a table. The computation of the whole is a function of how the individual parts are configured. Fields programmable gates arrays can be reprogrammed to the desired functionality requirements after manufacturing."[60]

In the living body, this reprogramming is a reconstruction processed through adaptation by the innate law. The computation involves construction, deconstruction and reconstruction of structural E/matter (Prin. 26) that constitute the adaptation of all the parts of the body for mutual benefit (Prin. 23).

The language of neurons and synapses (coded by the innate law) are connected to bodily functions.[61] Since it is impossible to give what we do not have, we can therefore only construct that which exists and can be copied in principle. For example, the universal Turing machine was constructed due to the property of biological copy-ability.

The innate law is really a 100%/perfect software processing data through an operating system, application programs, coders, device drivers, network interface, etc. Neurons are akin to computer hardware (CPU, transmitters, hardware platform interface, modulators, processors, microprocessors, decoders, receptors, feedback loop, etc.). Bodily functions are akin to the actions that a computer performs (taking data input, processing instructions, manifesting data output, etc.). This means that the computation of data (information/F) unites the software (organizing principle) with the manifestation of data (motion of E/matter) demonstrating the function of information/F (Prin. 10). If the body is a biological computer, then the physical brain is a biological central processing unit (CPU) and the nerves are a network system of transmitters. The nervous system is basically a sophisticated hardware system used to compute and transmit innate information/F, governed by the innate law, for coordination of actions of all the parts of the organism (Prin. 23, 32, 33).

ART. 253. INTERNAL INNATE CONSTRUCTION

It is difficult to see the physical brain and its nerves without preconceptions. "One innate impulse for every cell of the body" is falsified by the example of an organ transplant. A heart being transported is maintained alive in a special solution for several hours without a brain to centralize and nerves to transmit innate impulses. If we are to move forward, we must close our eyes, and open them back up as if we are seeing the nervous system for the very first time. To see the physical brain without those rules that lock us will help us to see something new. Therefore, to observe that the nerve system is the system through which the innate law centralizes and transmits innate impulses for coordination of action in animal bodies is to delve into the area where there can be interference with the momentum of transmission of information/F (Prin. 12, 29).

In order to explain this old observation in a new way, parallel logic must be utilized to facilitate the understanding of the induction. The maxim, "we cannot give what we do not have" is true. That is to say that whatever we "construct" into external structural forms is always a reflection of internal

60. Field Programmable Gate Array (FPGA) xilinx.com/products/silicon-devices/fpga/what-is-an-fpga.html (Jan 2021)

61. Synapse. The Encyclopaedia Britannica. Britannica.com/science/synapse (Jan 27, 2025)

living systems. This is due to the counterfactual property of copy-ability which means that unless it is possible to discover a new principle that can be copied in applying its rules, we cannot construct a new structural form that would be dependent on the new principle. For example, the discovery of the principle of aerodynamics with its properties of being copyable and applicable, enabled the construction of a new structural form, the aircraft. This explains clearly why the use any external educated constructs can be relied upon as being a reflection of internal innate constructs (birds, insects, bats, etc.). It is the reason why when we observe computer data processing systems, what we observe are external educated structures that truly reflect internal innate structures. For example, living, thinking E/matter already exists in the universe, on planet earth, and is alive in us (Prin. 1, 20, 23). It is a component of who we are as human beings. That is why we can construct and actualize architectures and technologies, due to the property of copy-ability of the many internal innate structures that constitute the body of a living thing. Examples abound, such asthe water pump (heart), bridges (ligaments), filter (nose), artificial breathing machine (lungs), camera (eye), telephone (ear), irrigation (circulatory system), data processing systems (brain and nerves), etc.

In the next flowchart, the metabolism of tissue cells, the coordination of activities of body parts, and the voluntary actions are demonstrated:

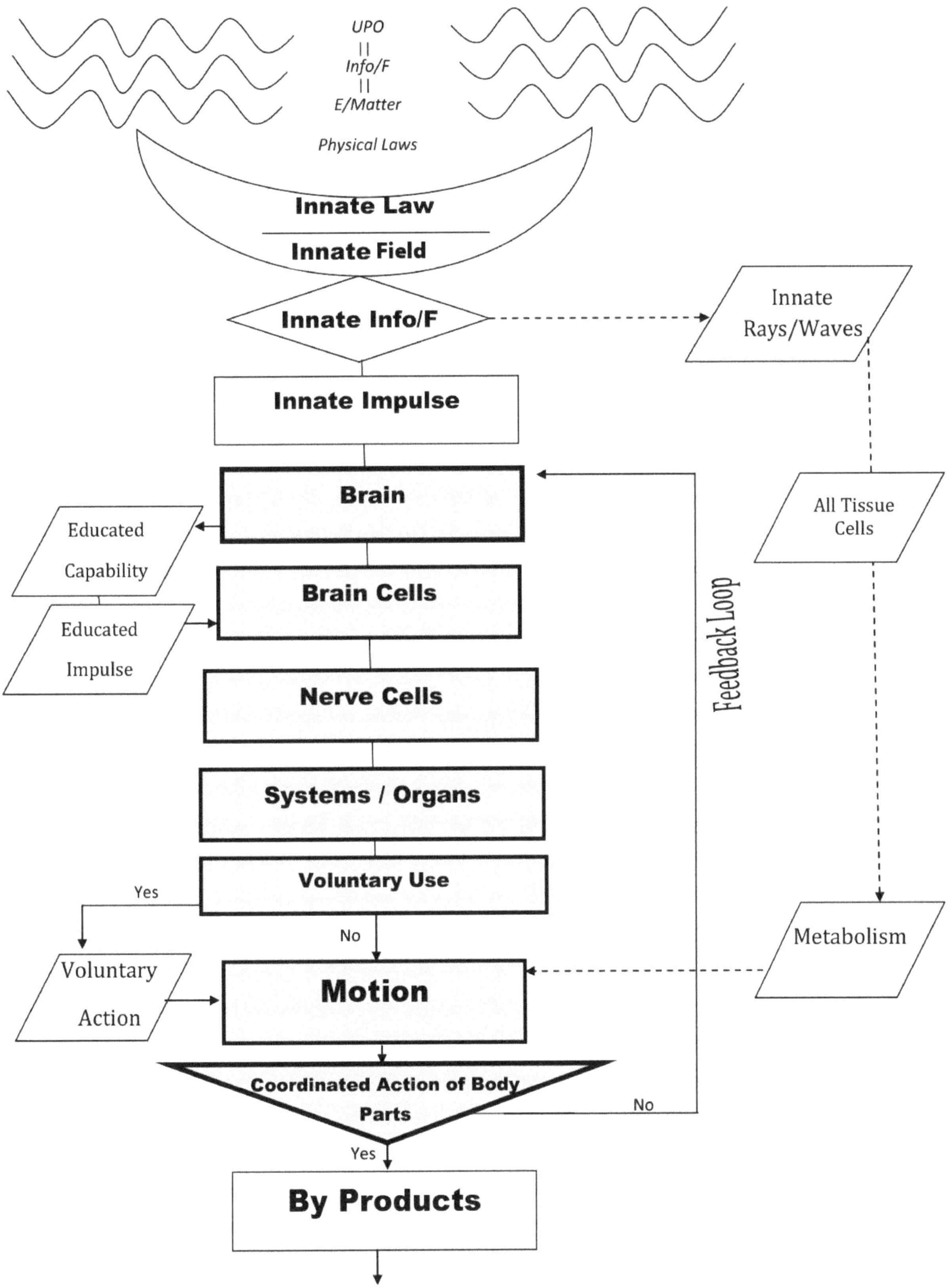

Fig. 33. Flowchart of the innate law within vertebrates. - Adaptation of information/Fand E/matter for bodily use via innate rays/waves for metabolism. Adaptation of information/F and E/matter for coordination of action via innate impulses. Adaptation of Information/F and E/matter and for voluntary actions via educated impulses, which are tinctured innate impulses.

ART. 254. CONSERVATION OF INFORMATION

Is information subject to the universal laws of conservation? The answer is an emphatic yes! "In the classical world, information can be copied and deleted at will. In the quantum world, however, the conservation of quantum information means that information cannot be created nor destroyed. This concept stems from two fundamental theorems of quantum mechanics: the no-cloning theorem and the no-deleting theorem". It was experimentally proven in 2007 by the discovery of the "no hiding theorem".[62] "Now for the first time, a team of physicists consisting of Pati, along with Jharana Rani Samal (deceased) and Anil Kumar of the Indian Institute of Science in Bangalore, India, has experimentally tested and confirmed the no-hiding theorem." The physicists, who performed all of the experimental work, have published their study on the no-hiding theorem test in a recent issue of Physical Review Letters.[63]

The "no-hiding theorem," addresses information loss in the quantum world. According to the "no-hiding theorem," if information is missing from one system (which may happen when the system interacts with the environment), then the information is simply residing somewhere else in the Universe. The missing information cannot be hidden in the correlations between a system and its environment. Physicists Samuel L. Braunstein at the University of York, UK, and Arun K. Pati of the Harish-Chandra Research Institute, India, first proved the "no-hiding theorem" in 2007. Until now, however, the "no-hiding theorem" had been a purely theoretical concept.[64]

This new knowledge introduces us to the extremely important new fact that information/F is subject to the universal laws of conservation and cannot be created nor destroyed. It is consistent with principle 5 revealing that the universe is 100%/perfect and complete as it states that: "In order to have existence, there must be 100%/perfect organizing principle, 100%/perfect information/force and 100%/perfect energy/matter."

ART. 255. NON-DISCRETE ASPECT OF INNATE IMPULSE (INSTRUCTION FUNCTION)

In 1953 Francis Crick, Rosalind Franklin, James Watson and Maurice Wilkins discovered the double helix of DNA. It provided insights into the genetic code. This code is information-based. From this discovery emerged the idea that the innate law of living things provided information/force to energy/matter to maintain bio-chemical balance. Every single characteristic of living E/matter is innate information/F, which has been adapted and computed by the innate law to maintain living E/matter alive according to universal laws (Prin. 21, 23, 24). Innate information/F is what makes living E/matter a more complex level of organization. DNA has the ability to be copied; it has copy-ability from generation to generation according to the limitation of E/matter.[65]

---

62. Zyga, Lisa. "Quantum No-hiding Theorem Experimentally Confirmed for First Time." Phys.org News (03/07/2011). https://phys.org/news/2011-03-quantum-no-hiding-theorem-experimentally.html (viewed 03/03/2025)

63. Jharana, Rani, Samal, et al. "Experimental Test of Quantum No-hiding Theorem." *Phys Review Letters. 106, 080401 (2011)* doi: *10.1103/PhysRevLett.106.080401*

64. Zyga, Lisa. "Quantum No-hiding Theorem Experimentally Confirmed for First Time." Phys.org News (03/07/2011). https://phys.org/news/2011-03-quantum-no-hiding-theorem-experimentally.html (viewed 03/03/2025)

65. DNA Replication. www.genome.gov/genetics-glossary/DNA-replication (03/03/2025)

A gene is the smallest unit of genetic information/F. It is a sequence of nucleotides within DNA. It gives the cell its biological identity within highly complex living organisms. This is a new model of innate information/F with its non-discrete (metaphysical) aspect. This is what chiropractic exclusively addresses, namely the interference in the momentum transmission of the innate impulse through the correction of vertebral subluxations.

The organization of the non-discrete aspect of innate information/F is computed and adapted by the essential extension of a universal principle of organization (Prin. 1) which bespeaks a universal intelligence. It is called the innate law of living things. Innate information/F is a non-discrete code of instructions to adapt living E/matter so that it is maintained alive according to universal laws (Prin. 21, 23, 24). The information aspect of the innate impulse is non-discrete (metaphysical). Codes of a computer program are bits of information. The physical aspect, hardware and wiring are simply transmitters of computed information. The computer codes must be programmed and organized to construct elaborate software that will run and govern the device. It takes organized coding and organized decoding processes that are programmed into the computer by the programmer in order to be of any value to the user. The same applies to the living body. It takes coded innate information/F for coordination of activities and decoded innate information/F for feedback under innate control.

All of our senses are sensors of universal information/F and E/matter that have been adapted by the innate law into innate sensory impulses that are transmitted through afferent nerves to the appropriate sector-decoder in the physical brain for interpretation.

REVIEW QUESTIONS FOR ARTICLES 251 - 255

1. Describe is the innate information/F action loop.
2. Why is the information action loop necessary in the body?
3. What is the type of innate information/F transmitted through the afferent pathway for coordination of activities?
4. What is required besides normal transmission of innate impulses for coordination of activities of body parts?
5. What is the meaning of interoperability through interconnectivity?
6. Using computer analogy, what is the 100%/perfect software in the body?
7. Using computer analogy, what is the operating system in the body?
8. Using computer analogy, what is the CPU in the body?
9. Using computer analogy, what are the transmitters in the body?
10. Describe the counterfactual property of "we cannot give what we do not own."
11. Is information subject to the universal laws of conservation?
12. What is the cause of the universal principle of organization?
13. What is the metaphysical aspect of the innate impulse?
14. What adapts the non-discrete (metaphysical) aspect of information/F?
15. Can the non-discrete (metaphysical) aspect of innate information/F be measured empirically?

ART. 256. DISCRETE ASPECT OF INNATE IMPULSE (FUNCTION OF MOMENTUM)

For existence to be maintained, all E/matter of the universe, including living E/matter, is organized at the atomic level from universal information/F (Prin. 1). In the living body, universal information/F is adapted, processed, computed, and coded into innate information/F for use in the body and for the coordination of action of all the body parts for mutual benefit and to keep the body alive according to universal laws (Prin. 21, 23, 24). Innate information/F is coded into innate impulses for coordination of activities, or into innate rays/waves for coherence of metabolism, or into innate trophic impulses/signals for feedback or innate sensory impulses for environmental adaptation. All of those impulses are coded by the innate law (100%/perfect software), which governs the living body (computer). Remember that you are not your body. You are more than your body. You lose an eye and you would still be you. Your body is the device that you use to navigate life circumstances and relate to its environment, including other human beings.

Since the living body is also comprised of E/matter, innate impulses must at some point manifest physicality. This process is the normal function of the innate law (Prin. 27), which is to adapt universal information/F and organize the construction (coding) and assembling of innate impulses which are then conducted through the nerve system in vertebrate animal bodies for coordination of activities and of innate rays/waves that are radiated from within each cell for metabolism. The function of neurons is to transmit time sensitive innate information/F for coordination of activities (Prin. 6, 23, 28). The innate impulse is a time sensitive message transmitted through conductive neurons to the body parts for coordination of activities. The innate impulse informs the body part as to what to do, in the moment, and how to act in coordination with all the other body parts for mutual benefit (Prin. 23). It is the physical nerve system, as conductor, that is the carrier of the time sensitive transmission of innate impulses. It is the physical transmission of the innate impulse as a physical impulse through the nerve system that is the physical aspect of the innate impulse. The non-physical aspect of the innate impulse cannot be measured empirically because, as an innate instruction, it is non-discrete. The physical aspect of the innate impulse can be measured empirically because, being physical, it is discrete.

In 1975 Chung Ha Suh, Ph.D., Seth Sharpless, Ph.D., and Marvin Luttges, Ph.D. conducted laboratory experiments at the Biomechanics Department of the University of Colorado that tested the effect of nerve root compression. The results revealed that as little as 10mm Hg of pressure (the weight of a U.S.A. dime) on a nerve root caused as much as 60% alteration in nerve function of that particular impinged physical nerve. The function of a neuron-transmitter is to transmit innate information/F in the form of impulses (innate, trophic, sensory and educated). This laboratory experiment verified that interference with the momentum of transmission of time sensitive innate impulse for coordination of activities occurs at the physical spinal nerve root and may be due to vertebral subluxation.[66] The innate-normal timing of the transmission of the innate impulse from physical brain to physical body part is paramount in order to satisfy the principle of coordination (Prin. 32). There is no such thing as a distorted instructive information/F for it is non-discrete. The interference issue is within the physical aspect of the innate impulse not the metaphysical aspect of the instruction. The message is always 100%/perfect and true (Prin. 5, 22, 27). It is the timing that is off (Prin. 6). It is directly an aspect of limitation of E/matter and time (Prin. 6, 24) since the vertebral subluxation furthers the limitation of E/matter through its interfering with the momentum in transmission of the innate impulse for coordination of activities. This means that for the body to have a timely flow of information/F, time is of the essence. As principle 29 states, "There can be interference in transmission of conducted innate

66. Sharpless, S.K., "Susceptibility of Spinal Nerve Roots to Compression Block." DHEW Publication (NIH) 767-998, (1975)

information/F." For example, if you had a scheduled exam at 10 am and you showed up at 11am, you would have missed the test and failed because you presented yourself at the wrong time. You studied, you know your material very well, and you got a failing grade. It is the same when an innate impulse with a specific code arrives at the wrong time due to interference in momentum of transmission caused by a vertebral subluxation that produced a lack of ease of the transmitting neurons because the tone of the nerve is too slack or too tense.[67] The result will be in-coordination of DIS-EASE (Prin. 30) and the principle of coordination will be violated (Prin. 32).

If there is an attenuation of the momentum of transmission of the innate impulse, due to vertebral subluxation, the instructive information/F will be received in an untimely manner (Prin. 28, 29, 30, 31). If any coordinative information/F is not received in a timely manner and the cause of the issue is not corrected, the activities of the organism are no longer coordinated. That is exactly what happens when a vertebral subluxation is present in the body (Prin. 31a). Vertebral subluxation is an interference that always causes a lack of ease of the transmitting neurons that alters the momentum in transmission of the innate impulse (Prin. 30, 31a). When the momentum in the transmission of the innate impulse is altered, it causes a lack of timing for the reception of the instructive information at the receptor body part, which violates the principle of coordination (Prin. 29, 32). This interference occurs within the physical aspect of the innate impulse. The location of this interference is at the impinged neuron-transmitters, which is then in a state of DIS-EASE (lack of ease), in which case, the nerve is too tense or too slack altering the momentum of the transmission of the innate impulse, thus causing an untimely instructive innate impulse at the receptor-body part for coordination of activities. The issue is the lack of innate-normal momentum (flow) of transmission of innate impulses (Prin. 6, 20). The integrity of the neuron-transmitters that are involved in the transmission of innate impulses is the exclusive focus of the chiropractic objective (Prin. 29, 30, 31a, 31b).

The non-discrete aspect of the innate impulse is united to the discrete aspect of the innate impulse through 100%/perfect instantaneous integral adaptation under innate control. This literally means that the adapted innate information/F for coordination of activities, by the innate law, instantaneously becomes an innate impulse as it is organized, coded and assembled (constructed) within the innate field of the physical brain (CPU) for centralized control.

Another adaptation of innate information/F is coded in to innate rays/waves for coherence of intra-cell particulates (components of the tissue cells) for metabolism of the organs, of the systems, and of the whole body. To help us understand what is really going on, we arbitrarily assign the innate law of the body, the innate law of the systems, the innate law of the organs, and the innate law of the tissue cells. For example, a heart transplant oftentimes requires the transportation of the organ, say from one location to another. The several hours spent from the removal the heart of the donor's body for transplant into the recipient's body was possible because the innate law of that particular organ, that was transported within a special solution within an organ care system, kept the heart alive without any innate impulses transmitted from the physical brain through the nerve system. It was processed by the innate law of the organ, as radiating innate rays/waves, from within the innate field of the organ, that instructed the intra-cell particulates of the heart itself, through adaptation, and kept it alive long enough for the transplant to be performed. In these cases, time is of the essence, usually under six hours. This is also only possible because the innate rays/waves are radiated for the coherence of the components of all the cells of the heart. Soundness of vitality through coherence of intra-cellular particulates of the organ is paramount for keeping living E/matter alive. Chiropractic does not address innate rays/waves. It is the

67. Palmer, D.D., "Text-Book of the Science, Art, and Philosophy of Chiropractic for Students and Practioners." Portland, OR: Portland Printing House Company. (1910) p.7

purpose of the innate law to maintain E/matter alive for a lifetime (Prin. 21) through its function, which is to adapt E/matter and information/F (Prin. 23), according to universal laws (Prin. 24).

ART. 257. INCOORDINATION

In-coordination is the lack of harmony of the actions of the body parts and a lack of coherence of soundness of body parts, due to an increase in the limitation of E/matter. The innate control, which is the activity of the innate law within the innate field, is always 100%/perfect and normal (Prin. 22, 27). The innate control functions only according to universal laws (Prin. 24).

The lack of coordination of activities is always due to a lack of ease (DIS-EASE) of the transmitting E/matter, directly or indirectly caused by a vertebral subluxation (Prin. 30, 31a). The activities of body parts are only coordinative if and only if there is an innate-normal momentum of transmission of innate impulses from physical brain (CPU) through the physical spinal nerves (transmitters) conforming to the principle of continuous supply and computation (Prin. 33). Coherence of soundness (vitality) of the body parts from body chemistry coursing through the serous circulation for metabolism and innate rays/waves radiating from within tissue cells of body parts providing coherence of cellular components is mandatory as well. Chiropractic addresses exclusively the correction of vertebral subluxation (Prin. 31).

ART. 258. LACK OF ADAPTATION

Lack of adaptation is the failure of the computation, codifying, processing and regulating of universal information/F within the tissue cell by the innate control because of the limitation of E/matter (Prin. 24). Interference in transmission of innate information/F (Prin. 29) further increases the limitation of E/matter, thereby decreasing its ability to be adaptable. That's exactly what the vertebral subluxation causes, the correction of which is the exclusive objective of chiropractic. The structural failure is always due to the limitation of E/matter. The innate law is limited by the limitation of E/matter (Prin. 24). It is the structural form of E/matter that is limited, not its atomic elements since those are never created nor destroyed (Prin. 5). The failure is never from the innate control or innate information/F because the innate law and its function are always perfect and normal (Prin. 22, 27). The purpose of innate information/F is innate balance of universal information/F, which is always in the tissue cells to maintain them in existence (Prin. 1, 14, 16). Lack of balance in the body lets un-adapted universal information/F, which are deconstructive toward structural E/matter (Prin. 26), act according to the un-adapted laws of physics or chemistry. Lack of balance in the body causes lack of internal resistance, thus leaving the body subject to concussion of universal information/force overcoming the internal resistance of the body. Innate balance in the body is limited by an altered momentum of transmission of innate impulses for coordination of activities. It is also limited by a lack of coherence between innate rays/waves from within the cells and body chemistry coursing through the serous circulation for soundness of cellular metabolism. Chiropractic addresses exclusively the correction of vertebral subluxation to restore normal transmission of innate impulses (Prin. 31a, 31b).

ART. 259. INSTRUCTIONS OF CHIROPRACTIC'S BASIC SCIENCE

The 33 principles of chiropractic's basic science are instructive information guiding the practice of the chiropractic objective. They consist of instructions transmitted to chiropractors in a timely manner. They must be critically studied with a view to falsify their veracity. It is crucial for the student to not accept those principles on faith and form a belief system of them. During the course of their chiropractic careers, chiropractors are constantly called to falsify the 33 principles of chiropractic's basic science, if they can. If they cannot, then the 33 principles of chiropractic's basic science are true until they can be falsified. Their conclusive revelation is exclusively the chiropractic objective to be practiced by chiropractors throughout the world to serve humanity. Therefore, when chiropractors follow the instructive information of the 33 principles of chiropractic's basic science and apply those principles, they instantly serve humanity. Chiropractic is a humanitarian approach to life in service to the wholeness of humanity.

ART. 260. CHIROPRACTIC'S BASIC SCIENCE UNITES CHIROPRACTIC PHILOSOPHY AND THE ART OF CHIROPRACTIC

Every field studies their specialized systems of principles that determine the field's objective in order to fulfill its purpose. Chiropractic is no exception. Chiropractic is constructed on a solid bedrock based on the instructive information of the 33 principles of its basic science, which reveals the chiropractic objective. Chiropractic philosophy is continually being developed as a hard to vary explanation of the 33 principles of chiropractic's basic science, which determine the chiropractic objective based on rational logic and deductive reasoning. Thus, it is through the application of those principles that the art of chiropractic is designed to practice the chiropractic objective in order to serve humanity. As long as we, together without condemnation, continue to follow diligently the instructions of the 33 principles of chiropractic's basic science, we can move forward without fear into a future of absolute confidence to practice the chiropractic objective.

For chiropractors to fulfill their mission, to stay on course and not deviate, they must meet two criteria. First, they must take responsibility to follow the guidance of the 33 principles of chiropractic's basic science in practice. Second, to fulfill its mission, the chiropractic profession must present and explain chiropractic as clearly as possible, over and over and over again, as many times as necessary, in as many ways as possible, to as many people as possible, so that humanity will have the best opportunity to choose to benefit from chiropractic care.

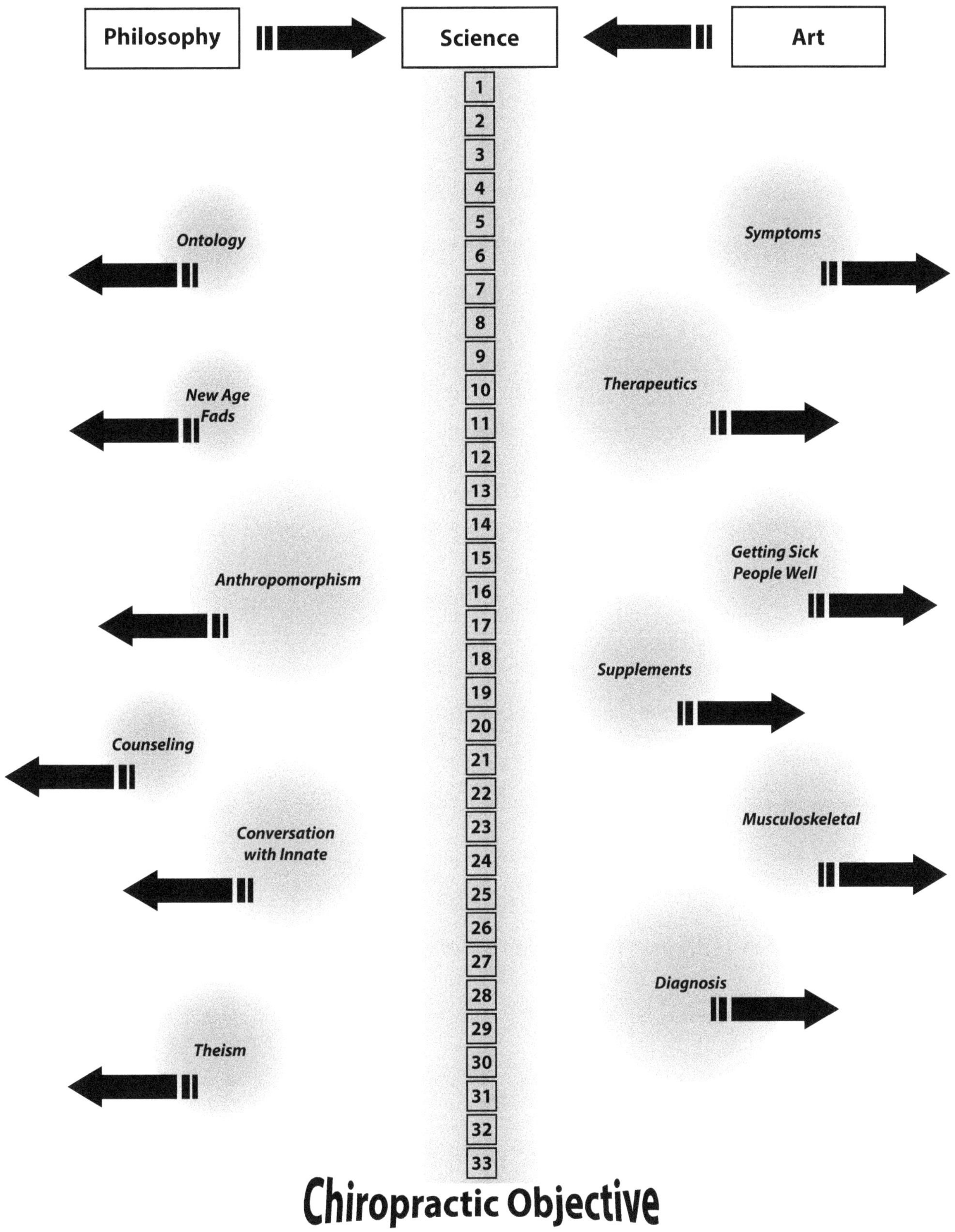

Fig. 34 is an illustration of the Guiding Principles Steering System (GPSS) for the practice of the chiropractic objective. Chiropractic philosophy is a hard to vary explanation of "WHY" the instructions of the 33 principles chiropractic's basic science are "WHAT" must be applied in order to know "HOW" to successfully make error corrections to stay on course to practice the chiropractic objective exclusively.

REVIEW QUESTIONS FOR ARTICLES 256 - 260

1. How many types of coded innate information/F are there in chiropractic?
2. Name the types of coded innate information/F.
3. What is the physical aspect of the innate impulse?
4. Can the physical aspect of the innate impulse be measured empirically?
5. When was it measured and what was the resultant conclusion?
6. Why is the momentum of the innate impulse so crucial to chiropractic?
7. How does the innate law maintain the body alive within the limitation of E/matter?
8. What is guiding the practice of the chiropractic objective?
9. What unites chiropractic philosophy with the art of chiropractic?
10. What two criteria must the chiropractic profession fulfill to accomplish its mission?
11. What is in-coordination?
12. What is the cause of in-coordination of activities in the body?
13. Does vertebral subluxation further increase the limitation of E/matter?
14. What is lack of adaptation?
15. What is the cause of structural failure of E/matter in the body?
16. Is the innate law of living things always 100%/perfect? Why?
17. What is the purpose of innate information/F in the body?
18. What is the only function that is always normal in the body?
19. What are the instructions of chiropractic's basic science?
20. What is it that unites chiropractic philosophy and the art of chiropractic?

ART. 261. NORMAL FUNCTION

According to the 33 principles of chiropractic's basic science the innate law is normal and its function is normal (Prin. 27). For a bodily function to be normal it must be what is called "innate-normal." This literally means that our educated intelligence is in no way capable to determine if a bodily function is normal or not normal. Only the 100%/perfect software (the innate law) is programmed in such a way that it can compute information/F and process tissue cells in order to adapt them for innate-normal function, moment to moment, if it is possible according to universal laws. The adaptability of E/matter is dependent upon its limitations. Thus, any bodily function is always limited and varies moment to moment, manifesting only innate-normal according to circumstances including the limits of adaptability. Remember the innate law is adapting information/F and E/matter within the limitations of E/matter and time (Prin. 6). It will adapt information/F and E/matter for the body only if it is possible according to universal laws (Prin. 24). What can be done? Practice the chiropractic objective exclusively, which is to locate, analyze, and facilitate the correction of vertebral subluxations for the innate-normal transmission of innate impulses.

ART. 262. INNATE-NORMAL

Innate-normal is one of the most important principles of chiropractic's basic science. To understand innate-normal, is essential to the practice of the chiropractic objective. According to the principles of chiropractic's basic science, the innate law and its function are what is always normal in the body all of the time (Prin. 27). The innate law will always perfectly adapt information/F and E/matter (Prin. 22, 23) if it is possible according to universal laws (Prin. 24). This means that regardless of circumstances, the perfect coordinative functions of the parts of the body will always occur within the limits of adaptation. This is why chiropractic concerns itself exclusively with the correction of vertebral subluxations because they further increase the limitations of E/matter by decreasing its adaptability. By practicing the chiropractic objective, which facilitates the correction of vertebral subluxations (Prin. 31b) chiropractors participate in the ongoing possibilities of increasing the adaptability of E/matter by decreasing the further limitations of E/matter caused by vertebral subluxations. The body instantly becomes more adaptable without vertebral subluxations. Therefore, body physiology is of no concern to chiropractors. The innate law will only adapt E/matter according to the limits of its adaptability if it is possible according to universal laws (Prin. 24). The innate law is truly limited by the limitation of E/matter. This is the core strength of chiropractic in a nutshell. Remove the interference to the momentum of transmission of innate impulses through the facilitation of the correction of vertebral subluxations (Prin. 31b) and you have done more than can ever be done for the continual evolutionary process of the species. By restoring the momentum of transmission of innate impulses to innate-normal, you participate in the "only" normal there is for the body. It is unique to the individual and varies moment to moment under specific circumstances. It's a matter of the individual body's adaptive ability to certain external or internal conditions. Only innate-normal is the norm for the living body. A clear understanding of innate-normal is paramount to practicing the chiropractic objective and to educate the practice members. The understanding of this important principle (Prin. 27) is the solid bedrock promoting ongoing regular chiropractic care for a lifetime.

Any attempt for the educated mind to know innate-normal is to simply make an educated guess. For the educated mind to try to determine what is normal the living body is presumptuous since normal adaptation from the living body varies moment to moment. To assume what is normal for a practice member is at best, arrogant, and at worst, fatal. With the knowledge we have accumulated over thousands of years, all of the world together without condemnation, we know so little of how the body must be adapted moment to moment.

In chiropractic there is an establishment of innate-normal standards. It is only by practicing exclusively the chiropractic objective that chiropractors recognize the individual's uniqueness and the ability of the living body to normalize itself, so long as there is no interference in transmission of innate impulses for coordination of activities, moment to moment.

ART. 263. ABNORMAL FUNCTION

According to the 33 principles of chiropractic's basic science, the only abnormal function in the body is a further increase in limitation of E/matter (Prin. 24) that is due, directly or indirectly, to the interference of transmission of innate information/F caused by vertebral subluxation (Prin. 29, 31). The lack of ease of the neuron-transmitters from the vertebral subluxation (Prin. 30) attenuates the momentum of transmission of innate impulses (Prin. 29), causing the reception of innate instructions to be received out of timing by the body part (Prin. 6). This untimely flow of information/F causes an untimeley reception of innate instructions from the body part. This is due to a vertebral subluxation, the result of which is an increased lack of adaptive ability of E/matter that causes in-coordination of activities of the whole body, which violates the principle of coordination (Prin. 32).

The further increase in limitation of E/matter from the interference in transmission of innate impulses will manifest something other than innate-normal. Only the 100%/perfect innate software can compute innate-normal adaptation of information/F and E/matter for use in the body, that continually vary moment by moment, so that all parts of the body will have coordinated action for mutual benefit according to the limitations of E/matter (Prin. 23, 24). Our educated intelligence, which is the capability of our educated brain to function, can only determine the presence of vertebral subluxation that causes the interference and address it accordingly to facilitate its correction. In chiropractic the only abnormal function in the body is a further increase in limitation of E/matter due, directly or indirectly to vertebral subluxations (Prin. 31a).

ART. 264. PARALYSIS IN CHIROPRACTIC

Paralysis is a body part that is lacking coordination of actions, or lacking soundness of tissue cells, or both. Paralysis is the tissue cell that has lost its innate-normal life. This tissue cell becomes dead to the innate law of the body. It may still be alive to itself through the innate law of the cell; however, it does not have coordinative actions to benefit the rest of the body. It only lives for itself. Paralysis is a state where living E/matter has reached the limits of its adaptability from the innate law for its coordinative purpose. From a chiropractic point of view, paralysis is the tissue cells of a body part that is disconnected from the coordinative activities of the rest of the body. It is no longer functioning for the mutual benefit of all the body parts. Its function is not innate-normal any longer. This is due to the further increase of the limitations of E/matter. Paralysis is an absolute. The tissue cell has either innate-normal functions or it has not.

ART. 265. LIFE AND DEATH

Life is innate-normal adaptation. Life is perfect coordination of activities of body parts. Life is soundness of tissue cells through innate-normal metabolism. In order to be maintained alive a tissue cell must be adapted by the innate law governing the cell, called the "innate law of the cell." For an organ it is the innate law of the organ. For a bodily system it is the "innate law of the system." For the whole body, it is the "innate law of the body" (Prin. 20, 21, 23). Those designations are arbitrary to help us understand the life processes that are involved. It is possible for an organ to be dead to the body and to be still alive. For example, when a vertebral subluxation is present and interferes with the neuron-transmitters, the momentum of transmission of innate impulses will be attenuated. Those neuron-transmitters are "dead" (useless) as regards to the body since they are not transmitting the innate impulses according to innate-normal any longer, as they are not coordinative in their actions. Yet, they are maintained alive by their own neuronal innate law. This will eventually cause the affected neuron-transmitters to die completely having no more cellular life due to the lack of coordination of activities of the whole body which further increases the limits of their adaptive ability. However, should the vertebral subluxation be corrected, by the innate law of the body through the processing of a vertebral adjustment, the neuron-transmitters are said once again to be "alive" (useful) to the body since they are coordinative in their action. It truly underscores the importance for chiropractors to exclusively practice the chiropractic objective.

Death is zero adaptation. Death is absence of coordination. Death is total lack of soundness of tissue cells in which E/matter of the body is only manifesting un-adapted universal information/F.

A comparison: 100% innate-normal adaptation is 100% life. 0% adaptation is 0% life; it is death. Somewhere in between is paralysis.

The 100%/perfect innate law is limited by the limitation of E/matter (Prin. 24). The innate law will adapt E/matter and information/F in coherence with circumstantial change, moment to moment. For this reason, chiropractors who choose to practice the chiropractic objective participate in the removing the further limits of adaptation of E/matter caused by vertebral subluxations.

REVIEW QUESTIONS FOR ARTICLES 261 – 265

1. What is normal function?
2. What is innate-normal?
3. What further increases the limitations of E/matter in the living body?
4. What is it that decreases the adaptability of living E/matter?
5. What is the only norm for the living body?
6. Is chiropractic concerned with body functions?
7. What is the core strength of chiropractic in a nutshell?
8. Can the educated mind know what is innate-normal?
9. How does chiropractic establish innate-normal standards?
10. Is there actually such a thing as abnormal function in the body?
11. What is abnormal function in the body?
12. What is paralysis in chiropractic?
13. Can a tissue cell be dead to the body (useless) and still be alive to itself?
14. Why is paralysis an absolute in chiropractic?
15. In chiropractic, what is life?
16. In chiropractic, what is death?
17. In death, what is the state of E/matter?

ART. 266. CAUSE OF PARALYSIS IN CHIROPRACTIC

The function of E/matter is the expression of information/F organized by the universal principle of organization (Prin. 13). The function of the innate law of living things is to adapt both information/F and E/matter for use in the body (Prin. 23). The innate law is a 100%/perfect software that adapts E/matter through computation, processing and coding universal information/F into innate impulses, innate rays/waves, innate trophic impulses/signals, innate sensory impulses, and educated "tinctured" innate impulses. Chiropractic addresses exclusively innate impulses for coordination of activities. This adaptation is continuous and varies moment to moment according to the internal and external circumstances of the body (Prin. 33). Therefore, interference in the momentum of transmission of innate impulses (Prin. 29) from a lack of ease (DIS-EASE) or tone of the neuron-transmitters of the nerve which is too slack or too tense (Prin. 30), due to vertebral subluxation (Prin. 31), will violate the principle of coordination (Prin. 32). As a result, communication between the E/matter of the physical brain and the E/matter of the body part is altered, thus causing paralysis of coordinative actions of the entire body, which is called incoordination of actions. While the innate impulse is always perfect, the expression of its innate instruction to E/matter will be ever changing because the internal and external environmental conditions are ever changing. The lack of ease (DIS-EASE) of the neuron-transmitters, which is a lack of tone caused by a vertebral subluxation, alters the transmission first, of its own innate impulses, resulting in improper actions of the nerve system to conduct the innate information/F to the body parts. This is due to alteration of living E/matter, which is a further increase of its limits of adaptation. It is less adaptable. The problem is always within discrete E/matter. It is never a problem of the non-discrete 100%/perfect innate law. It just so happens that, according to the principles of chiropractic's basic science, the innate law of living things will not break a universal law (Prin. 24).

ART. 267. ENVIRONMENTAL VARIABLES.

Environmental variables are the environment of the organism that is continually in a state of flux, ever changing. The innate impulse is always 100%/perfect and normal (Prin. 22, 27). The expression of that perfect innate impulse will be in flux as well and will vary according to the circumstances of the particular moment. The living body is constantly in flux through cellular replacement at the rate of 330 billion cells per day. Only the innate law, which adapts all information/F and E/matter, can process this flux at the perfect level of innate-normal. It is called 100%/perfect instantaneous integral adaptation. Depending upon the limitations of E/matter, the innate law will compute, moment to moment, exactly what is present for processing, as long as the momentum of transmission of innate impulses for coordination of activities and of radiation of innate rays/waves for soundness of tissues are innate-normal. Chiropractic addresses exclusively the vertebral subluxations which is an interference in momentum of transmission of innate impulses that causes a lack of ease (DIS-EASE) of the neuron-transmitters affecting nerve tone (too slack or too tense) which leads to in-coordination of activities of body parts, thus violating the principle of coordination (Prin. 29, 30, 31, 33).

ART. 268. COMPENSATORY ADAPTATION

Compensatory adaptation is computation of information/F and E/matter by the innate law, due to the lack of coordinative activities of a body part, for the purpose of keeping the whole body in coherence, if it is possible according to universal laws (Prin. 24, 33). It occurs through 100%/perfect instantaneous integral adaptation. This literally means that the innate-normal adaptation of all the tissue cells of the all the body parts will be integrated to keep the whole body in balance. It underscores the importance for all chiropractors to practice the chiropractic objective exclusively. Chiropractic is a humanitarian evolutionary approach to life, of all of life experiences with no exception.

ART. 269. ADAPTABILITY OF E/MATTER

A wide range of ever more sophisticated complex properties and actions of E/matter and universal information/F can be observed. These properties demonstrate highly organized manifestations that give rise to the ability of E/matter to be adaptable, a differentiation of E/matter between non-living E/matter and living E/matter. There is a fundamental and universal scientific organizing principle that is operating at every level of organization to maintain E/matter in existence, and at times, to maintain it alive for a while within its genetic lifespan limitations. It is due to the adaptability of E/matter caused by the innate law of living things, which is an essential extension of the universal principle of organization, to govern living E/matter. The innate law maintains the body of a living thing alive within its limitations according to universal laws (Prin. 24).

Within these different levels of organization, the essential extension of the organizing principle called the innate law of living things adapts, computes, and codes universal information/F to construct even more complex organizations of E/matter giving rise to living E/matter. This newly-coded information/F transforms and constructs atoms into molecules, molecules into compounds, and compounds into living tissue cells for use in the body. These new structural forms of E/matter are constructed and governed by what is now called the innate law of living things. As a result of this new adapted universal information/F and E/matter, there is a new re-formation or re-construction of the structural forms of E/matter that is now manifesting signs of life, one being adaptability (Prin. 18). The innate law is investing a new character-code to E/matter, transforming the properties and actions of E/ matter into active-living organization (living E/matter.) This new adapting, controlling, and balancing law is called the "innate law of living things" and it is intrinsic exclusively to living E/matter. Therefore, this innate law adapts and balances universal information/F and E/matter to maintain it alive based on principle 1 that maintains all E/matter in existence.

ART. 270. LACK OF ADAPTABILITY OF E/MATTER

All structural E/matter is limited. It is only at the level of the atom that E/matter is most stable as it is conserved and maintained in existence through its properties and actions from the universal principle of organization (Prin. 1). The universe is complete (Prin. 5). At the complex level of living things, structural E/matter demonstrates one of the signs of life namely, adaptability, which is pre-determined from its genetic code, called the DNA. From the onset of its construction, living E/matter manifests genetic limitations through specific properties and actions. For example, a polar bear will sustain arctic cold of -40°F while tropical heat of 120°F will kill it. On the other hand, a lion from Africa will sustain tropical heat of 120°F while arctic cold of -40°F will kill it. There is a specific limit of adaptability within all living tissues. This is due the law of genetics with its genetic limitations. This also means all living tissues possess an innate-normal genetic adaptability that cannot be more than its pre-determined genetic code. It is a universal law. The student is reminded that the only normal function is the function of the innate law (Prin. 27). That is why the innate law adapts information/F and E/matter of the body and only if it is possible according to universal laws (Prin. 24) which includes the law of genetics. Chiropractic's basic science states that there can be interference in the transmission of conducted innate information/F (Prin. 29) through a lack of ease (DIS-EASE) of the neuron-transmitters which causes the tone of the nerve to be too slack or too tense due to vertebral subluxations (Prin. 30, 31a), which will further increase the limitations of E/matter. This in turn will cause a decrease of adaptability of the body part that will violate the principle of coordination (Prin. 32). According to the 33 principles of chiropractic's basic science, there can be only one abnormal function in the body, and that is a lack of adaptability of the body due the limitations of E/matter (Prin. 24). That is the only malfunction that chiropractors aim to address through the practice of the chiropractic objective. It is the vertebral subluxation that causes interference in the transmission of the momentum of innate impulses (Prin. 29, 30, 31a). This interference further increases the limitations of living E/matter, thereby decreasing the adaptability of living E/matter.

The student is reminded that the cause of vertebral subluxations is an external invasive information/F overcoming the internal resistance of the body. Internal resistance is directly dependent upon the adaptability of all the tissue cells of all the parts of the whole body. This means that there are several causes of lack of adaptability of E/matter. Chiropractic addresses exclusively one of them, which is the vertebral subluxation.

REVIEW QUESTIONS FOR ARTICLES 266 - 270

1. What is the cause of paralysis in chiropractic?
2. Is the lack of communication between the principle of organization and E/matter?
3. Is the lack of communication between the principle of organization and information/F?
4. Is the lack of communication between E/matter and E/matter?
5. Explain 100%/perfect instantaneous integral adaptation.
6. What is compensatory adaptation?
7. What is the purpose of compensatory adaptation?
8. What is the essential extension of the universal principle of organization called?
9. What is the most stable level of E/matter? Why?
10. What determines innate-normal adaptability?
11. In chiropractic, what is the one and only malfunction that exist in the body?
12. Which exclusive cause of further increased of the limitation of E/matter does chiropractic address?
13. What is the cause of a vertebral subluxation?
14. What is the internal body resistance dependent upon?

ART. 271. EDUCATED VERSION OF THE BRAIN

The educated version of the brain is a philosophical concept in chiropractic. It is that part of the brain used by the innate law of living things, as an organ, for reason, memory, education, conscience and the so-called voluntary actions, including the will. The educated brain is supplied with innate impulses by the innate law. It is liable to interference in momentum in transmission, thus it can have in-coordination of action. It is not vital. It is located within the gray E/matter which is mostly within the cerebral cortex of the brain but also throughout the whole body. It is the chief organ of adaptation to environmental conditions.

The educated brain is a variation of the physical brain. It is an organ used by the innate control for several specific purposes just as the liver and stomach are used for certain purposes. It is constructed of living E/matter, and therefore has limitations (Prin. 24). Thinking, intuition, instinct, intellectual processing of computation, reasoning, memory storage, retrieval, environmental perceptions and assessments are all subject to interference. They exist through the tincturing of innate impulses into educated impulses for conscious voluntary actions that pertains to the will. They can breakdown due to a multitude of causes. Chiropractic only addresses one cause: vertebral subluxation, which interferes with the momentum of transmission of innate impulses for coordination of activities of body parts (Prin. 29, 30, 31, 32). The practice of chiropractic is nothing more, nothing less and nothing else.

With regards to tincturing of innate impulses for voluntary actions, it is a capability of the educated brain of the individual (educated intelligence) to imbue a specific character of their resolve, to an innate impulse that transforms it into an educated impulse to perform a certain voluntary act. The original innate impulse is an adapted, characterized, and coded universal information/F by the innate law, which is then imbued by the educated intelligence through the educated brain with a specific new character-code. The innate impulse is modified into a coded educated impulse for voluntary actions that include memory, thinking, reasoning, intellectuality, consciousness, will, judgment, and learning. Educated impulses are tinctured innate impulses by the educable intelligence of the individual.

Therefore, the educated brain possesses a capability to function consisting of a learned versatility that can tincture innate impulses that will carry out voluntary actions. It is called "educated intelligence."

Note: The student is reminded that the universal principle of organization is the initial fundamental chiropractic principle that is organizing information/F providing properties and actions to all E/matter to be maintained in existence. Information/F may be adapted by the innate law into innate impulses for coordination of activities of all the parts of the living body. It may be adapted into innate rays/waves for metabolism for all the cells of the body by the innate law as well. Innate impulses can also be tinctured by the individual's resolve, utilizing his/her educated intelligence through the educated brain for voluntary actions.

ART. 272. EDUCATED INTELLIGENCE

Article 267 mentioned that only the innate law, which adapts all information/F and E/matter, can process everything at the perfect level of innate-normal. Educated intelligence is the capability of the educated brain to function. Chiropractic philosophy, through its unique lexicon, divides the brain into two fields that are acting as operating systems within the living body: the innate field of the central processing unit of the physical brain is the main operating system. The educated field of the educated brain is a sub-operating system. Both fields are completely governed by the innate law, with the exception that the educated brain possesses the capability (educated intelligence) to tincture the innate impulses that are assembled in the innate field of the gray E/matter of the brain and of the whole body into educated impulses for voluntary actions that includes reason, thinking, memory, education, conscience, and the will. The interface of innate impulses and educated impulses is the educated field of the educated brain where the tincturing from educated intelligence is processed. These educated impulses first pass through the innate field of the E/matter of the physical brain and of the whole body. Both fields are non-discrete and differentiated through their functions. The innate field is where innate impulses are assembled for coordination of activities and the educated field is where educated impulses are tinctured for voluntary actions. All of the tissue cells of the body are governed by the innate law through adaption of universal information/F and E/matter for use in the body (Prin. 23). There is no governance from educated intelligence, only usage for voluntary actions. For example, the educated intelligence does not govern the organ of sight; it simply employs the eyes to see where it wants to go for its own personal resolve. Only the innate law governs the organ of sight with all that it entails.

The innate field of the body is basically the operating system where the innate law constructs innate information/F into specific instructions for use in the body to maintain the body alive according to universal laws (Prin. 21, 22, 23, 24). The innate field is the space where the organizing principle and E/matter interface through the reorganization of information/F by the innate law. The innate field is everywhere in the body because the innate law of living things is everywhere in the body. It is literally everywhere the life of every tissue cell is maintained according to their limitations.

The innate field of the physical brain (CPU) is the operating system used by the innate law of living things to adapt universal information/F, and from that field, to codify and assemble innate impulses for coordination of activities. The educated field of the educated brain is a sub-operating system of the physical brain used by the educated intelligence to tincture and modify the innate impulse into an educated impulse for voluntary actions. The educated brain is located somewhere within the E/matter of the physical brain and of the whole body which is utilized by the innate law as a major organ of adaptation to the external environment of the organism. The educated intelligence, as a capability, can access the educated brain in order to adapt the body to outside circumstances and influences. For example, if you are cold outside, your educated intelligence makes use of your educated brain and you choose to go inside where it is warm or to put on a coat that will protect you from the cold. If you want to go to the store to buy something, you employ your educated intelligence to hop in your car and you drive there. If you want to learn chiropractic, you access your educated intelligence to enroll in a chiropractic college that teaches the philosophy, the science, and the art of chiropractic, and so on. Functioning as an organ, the educated brain has limitations of E/matter, like any other organ, and is subject to interference in transmission of innate information/F including the educated intelligence, which is the capability of the educated brain to function. The educated brain is a tangible, physical version of the brain and its capability to function is the educated intelligence.

ART. 273. EDUCATED CONTROL

Article 267 mentioned that only the innate law could perfectly process all the biological data of the body at the perfect level of innate-normal. The innate law is 100%/perfect innate software that runs the body by adapting all information/F and E/matter that is computed through perfect innate control, which is the activity of the innate law within the innate field of the whole body, including the physical brain moment to moment continuously (Prin. 33). Educated control is the activity of the innate law within the innate field of the educated body including the educated brain as an organ. The product of this activity is called thoughts for voluntary actions, such as reasoning, will, memory, movements, etc. It is always the innate law that adapts information/F and E/matter, for use in the body, including the voluntary organs and systems (Prin. 23). At times, innate impulses will be tinctured by the educated intelligence through the educated brain for voluntary actions (*See Fig. 4*). For example, it is important to note that we do not know how to operate the special sense organs even though we can will them to act. The operations of the sense organs are from the innate control. However, their functional use is from the educated control. Educated information/F is mostly for adaptation to the environment and is called "educated impulses." Educated impulses are innate impulses that have been tinctured (modified) by the educated intelligence for voluntary actions. It is the innate law that governs all data processing of the body. The educated intelligence can only make use, through tincturing, of some of the already computed innate impulses of the body by the innate control for voluntary actions.

The student is reminded that the living body can only be maintained alive by being adapted through the instructive information/F computed and coded by the innate law (Prin. 21, 23).

ART. 274. NON-MATERIAL REALITIES

At this point, it is necessary to discuss some fundamental understanding, according to what we know in the 2020s, of non-material realities. First of all, the initial condition of chiropractic's basic science is a universal principle of organization that is intrinsic to all E/matter (Prin. 1). Without it, E/matter would not be maintained in existence. The universal principle of organization is non-material; it is a fundamental organizing principle, which is the principle that continually maintains E/matter in existence. The function of the universal principle of organization is to organize information/F (Prin. 8). This fundamental principle organizes unlimited information/F maintaining all E/matter in existence. Therefore, living E/matter is also maintained in existence by this fundamental principle. The body of a living thing is governed by the innate law of living things, which maintains it alive (Prin. 20) if it is possible according to universal laws (Prin. 24). This innate law has been called, "the law of life," by B.J. Palmer, D.C.. Its function is to assemble universal information/F, adapt it by investing it with new character-codes and reorganizing it into innate information/F for all the tissue cells. We must remember that the innate law of living things can adapt an unlimited supply of universal information/F. The innate law is a part of the universal principle of organization, in so far as the universal principle is intrinsic to the existence of all E/matter including living things in the entire universe. The innate law is also apart from the universal principle of organization, in so far as the innate law is localized only within the physical structure of the body of individual living things, and is never localized within the physical structures of non-living things. The innate law is an essential extension (part of and part from) the universal principle of organization (comparable to a sun ray that is a part of and a part from the sun). The innate law is a localized aspect of the universal principle of organization, and as such, it is "under" the rule of the initial universal principle. As an example, Newton's third law of equal and opposite reaction is "under" the rule of his second law of acceleration of the law of gravity.[68] The innate law is non-material and maintains the body alive (Prin. 21). It is an essential extended continuation of the universal principle of organization that is also non-material and maintains all E/matter in existence (Prin. 1). The universal principle of organization is everywhere in the universe and the innate law of living things is everywhere within all living E/matter in the universe. The universal principle of organization and the innate law of living things are non-material and they are essentially one and the same. The innate law is simply the universal principle adapting more complex levels and states of E/matter. They are arbitrarily differentiated as universal principle of organization and innate law of living things for our own understanding. It is the same way

68. Densmore, Dana (ed.), "Selections from Newton's Principia" USA:GreenCat Books an imprint of Green Lion Press. (2004) p.31

when the law of universal gravitation and the law of geometry are differentiated, when they are truly one and the same.

"Einstein's general relativity is a mathematically beautiful application of geometric ideas to gravitational physics."[69] It is true due to the fact that the universal principle of organization has the property of copy-ability, which means that any other universal law is a simple copy of the original start point of chiropractic's basic science which is its initial condition, namely the major premise (Prin. 1).

ART. 275. ONE NORMAL FUNCTION RESTORING ONE ABNORMAL FUNCTION

In chiropractic there is only one normal function within the body of living things. It is the function of the innate law of living things (Prin. 27). Its function is to adapt universal information/F and E/matter for use in the body, so that all parts of the body will have coordinated actions for mutual benefit (Prin. 23). Adapted innate information/F are called innate impulses for coordination of activities, trophic impulses/signals for feedback from body part-receptor to brain-CPU, innate rays/waves for the governance of intra-cell particulates for metabolism, and sensory impulses for sensory organs of adaptation to external environment. Chiropractic is exclusively concerned with vertebral subluxation, an interference in transmission of innate impulses for coordination of activities. The conductor of innate impulses is the nerve system (Prin. 28). There can be interference with the momentum of transmission of innate impulses (Prin. 29) caused by a lack of ease of the neuron-transmitters (Prin. 30), in which the tone of the nerve is too slack or too tense, that directly or indirectly is due to vertebral subluxations (Prin. 31) thus, violating the principle of coordination (Prin. 32).

In practice, chiropractic applies the principle of the vertebral adjustment by the innate law (Prin. 31b) through the location, analysis and facilitation of the correction of vertebral subluxations in order to once again satisfy the principle of coordination (Prin. 32). It is as simple as that.

The definition of a vertebral subluxation is the condition of a vertebra that has lost its proper juxtaposition with the one above or the one below, or both; to an extent less than a luxation; which impinges nerves and interferes with the transmission of innate impulses.[70] All the factors of the foregoing definition must be given to define exactly what a vertebral subluxation is and to make it a, hard to vary, chiropractic explanation; nothing more, nothing less, nothing else.

When a vertebral subluxation occurs, the impingement upon the nerve induces a lack of ease (DIS-EASE) of some neuron-transmitters, which is the tone of the nerve being too tense or too slack, that alters the momentum of transmission of the innate impulses, which arrive at the body part-receptors "out of timing." The instructive information that the innate impulses carry is now received by the body part-receptor as an untimely flow of information/F. All processes require time (Prin. 6). The altered momentum of transmission of the innate impulses impedes the decoding and computation of the time sensitive instructive information at the receptor site and will bring about in-coordination of DIS-EASE (Prin. 30), which violates the principle of coordination (Prin. 32). When the lack of ease (DIS-EASE) of the neuron-transmitters happens, it further increases the limitation of E/matter (Prin. 24) due to the interference in the transmission of the innate impulse. The living E/matter of the whole body is more limited and is less adaptable for coordination of activities (Prin. 18, 23).

69. Ashtekar, Berger, Isenberg, and MacCallum (eds.) "Gravity is Geometry, after all. General Relativity and Gravation: A Centennial Perspective." Cambridge: Cambridge University Press. (2015) p. 347 doi: 10.1017/CB09781139583961.010

70. Stephenson, R.W., "Chiropractic Text Book." (Vol XIV) Davenport, IA: The Palmer School of Chiropractic. (1948) p. 2, 320

Through rational logic, deductive reasoning concludes that, from a chiropractic perspective, there is only one abnormal function in the whole body. It is a lack of adaptability of E/matter due to a further increase of its limitations. Chiropractic exclusively addresses the vertebral subluxation, which from its own definition above, "interferes with the transmission of innate impulses" that further increases the limitations of E/matter, thereby decreasing its ability to be adaptable by the innate law.

REVIEW QUESTIONS FOR ARTICLES 271 - 275

1. What is the educated version of the brain?
2. What is the educated brain?
3. What is the function of the educated brain?
4. Is the educated brain subject to in-coordination of action?
5. What is educated intelligence?
6. What is an innate impulse and what is its function?
7. What is an educated impulse and what is its function?
8. What is the innate field? Where is it located?
9. What is the educated field? Where is it located?
10. What is innate control?
11. What is educated control?
12. Explain the distinction between the universal principle of organization and the innate law of living things?
13. In chiropractic, what is the one and only normal function of the living body?
14. In chiropractic, what is the one and only abnormal function of the living body?

ART. 276. CHIROPRACTIC IS POSSIBLE ONLY ACCORDING TO UNIVERSAL LAWS

Universal laws are derived from fundamental, immutable, and perpetual truths. It is an invariable set of information/F that dictates the form and order of everything that exist which is derived from the universal principle of organization to maintain everything in existence. They are also called natural laws. They give constancy to the universe and its content. For example, they are manifested as the law of gravity, the law of thermodynamics, the law of aerodynamics, the law of conservation of E/matter, the law of genetics, etc.

Universal laws provide order and they are all derived from a fundamental universal principle of organization. Most people take these laws for granted. For example, do you ask why a rosebush blossoms as a rosebush and not into tulips or lillies? No, you don't. One rarely thinks about universal laws as they count on their incessant works. These laws provide information/F to the universe to maintain order.

All universal laws stem from a universal principle of organization, which is appropriated by chiropractic as the initial condition of chiropractic's basic science. All universal laws are information/F organized by the universal principle of organization and are intrinsic to all E/matter providing it with properties and actions that are expressed by E/matter to maintain it in existence (Prin. 1, 13). Information/F is the interface between the universal principle of organization and E/matter (Prin. 10).

Universal laws have always existed since the beginning of the Universe. They have been discovered over time. For example, Isaac Newtown discovered the law of gravitation in the 1600s. Then came Albert Einstein in 1905 who demonstrated that Newton's law of conservation of energy is valid. His equation $E=mc^2$ revealed that energy is the mass of matter at the speed of light squared. Einstein discovered that energy and matter are equivalent and interchangeable. In chiropractic it is called E/matter and it shows that force, in chiropractic, is not energy but information, hence the term information/F. It was in 1927 that Ralph Stephenson, D.C. described the innate law of living things (formally known as innate intelligence), which is an essential extension of the universal principle of organization. Furthermore, since a principle is a fundamental truth that is the foundation of universal laws, it clarifies the initial condition of chiropractic's basic science as being the foundation of all universal laws. All universal laws are caused by the universal principle of organization (Prin. 1) because universal laws are the epitome of organization to maintain universal order even though they may sometimes seem like chaos to us.

What is perceived through one's senses is not always accurate. For example, when I fly my airplane, I do not ignore the law of gravitation. On the contrary, I used the laws of aerodynamics with its subsets of thrust, lift, drag, airfoil and power to fly an object that is heavier than air. If I have enough fuel and I maintain the proper airspeed including the angle of attack, I will move from point A to point B following aviation vectors. All this happens because objects have mass and weight that attract each other. The airplane is capable of flying due to the lift that is generated by the thrust of the propeller, that is activated by the power of the engine, which is moving the flow of air to overcome the forces of the gravitational field in order to keep the aircraft airborne. This flight is only for a determined amount of time, of course, since eventually I will have to land my airplane to refuel so I can reach my destination safely. Every aircraft model has its own engineered functional limitations.

Interestingly enough the discovery of the law of aerodynamics by the Wright brothers and the discovery of the innate law of living things by D.D. Palmer occurred at the turn of the 20th century just a few years after the invention of the electric light bulb in 1879 by Thomas Edison. As our educated intelligence evolves, so is our understanding of universal laws that were beyond the grasp and imagination of our predecessors before the 1800s. Evolutionary thinking trusts the field of the future and holds the present with what we know up till now. Evolutionary thinking accepts knowing what we know at this moment while accepting that we don't know yet that which will be only known later in time (Prin. 6).

ART. 277. THE LIMITATIONS OF E/MATTER

Everything that exists in the universe functions according to universal laws. All E/matter functions according to universal laws, including living E/matter. Our bodies and minds are finite. Therefore, one cannot understand infinity. We cannot understand a universal intelligence that designed a universal principle of organization which we do not understand. It is a paradox. However, in chiropractic we assert that a universal principle of organization maintains all E/matter in existence with order and firmness (Prin. 1). It is the starting point of chiropractic's basic science.

E/matter is generally defined as anything that has weight and occupies space. There are many different kinds of E/matter. The periodic table reveals the elements that are known to science at the moment. More potentially exist, that have not been discovered yet. Depending on their specific properties and actions provided by the universal principle of organization, we can predict their behavior under certain circumstances. For example, we know that the universal principle of organization provides H_2O with the property and actions of being fluid in a temperature range of 33°-211°F, through the organizing of information/F (the configurations and velocities of electrons, protons, and neutrons). If we add heat, raising the temperature to 212°F, the universal principle of organization will provide H_2O with the property and action of being gas, through a different organizing of information/F. If we reduce temperature to 32°F, the universal principle of organization will provide H_2O with the property and actions of a solid, through yet another different organizing of information/F. These transformations are all explained through the universal principle of organization that reconfigures electrons, protons and neutrons of E/matter. The actual maintaining of existence of E/matter is defined by properties and actions provided by a universal principle of organization that governs E/matter according to universal laws. E/matter has its limitations (Prin. 24). At more complex levels of organized E/matter, life springs up with its sign of adaptability to give living E/matter the ability to be adaptable in accordance to universal laws (Prin. 18, 24).

The living body has its limitations. It lives for a while and passes away due its limitations, one of which is its longevity that results from the universal law of genetics. The body of living things cannot live forever. The body is limited in its capability to be adapted by the innate law. For example, if we cut a finger, the innate law through cellular replacement will heal the finger. If the finger is cut off completely, the innate law will most likely not be able through cellular replacement to regrow that finger. Cellular replacement occurs according to universal laws. As a matter of fact, life occurs according to universal laws. This is the reason that chiropractic is always about what is possible according to universal laws (Prin. 24).

ART. 278. LIMITATIONS OF TIME

The capability of the innate law to adapt information/F and E/matter for use in the body (Prin. 23) is limited by time because all processes require time (Prin. 6).

The new knowledge of $E=mc^2$ reveals how difficult it is to understand the concept of time. Even though we have the equation $t = d/s$, the standard theories of the unified field do not currently address the issue. What we know is that objects behave in ways that show time to be a different kind of dimension pertaining to the motion of E/matter through space. Time is a mathematical continuity where it advances smoothly in flow.[71] This simply means that time is related to space in the universe. It is space/time emerging from the universal principle that organized information/F to configures the subatomic particles of E/matter and their velocities in order to provide motion to E/matter to maintain it in existence (Prin. 1, 6, 8, 10, 13, 14, 15).

Even though Einstein's equation further developed Newton's view of time "flowing uniformly" and called "duration by means of motion",[72] it must be noted that E/matter exists as a result of its properties and actions being supplied by the universal principle of organization (Prin. 1).

All E/matter manifests motion (Prin. 14). This implies that E/matter, through the configuration and velocities of its electrons, protons, and neutrons, occupies space moving through time (Prin. 6). The motion of the particles of E/matter covers distance within space that can be measured and quantified in time (F = ma.) It is becoming clear why Stephenson mentioned, "Time is an element necessary to the bond between intelligence and matter".[73] This reveals a new equation in the form of, E/matter = Space/time. The "E" and the "m" of $E = mc^2$ are now just items to go on one side of the "=" sign linking them.[74] In the equation, E/matter = Space/time, the "=" sign is the organized of information/F by the universal principle of organization (Prin. 1, 3, 4, 8, 10, 13).

What is the bond between the organizing principle and E/matter? It is the second factor of the triune, namely, the non-discrete information/F. It is information/F that is the continuous interface or bond uniting the organizing principle to E/matter (Prin. 10). Therefore, we observe that within space, time is intrinsic to E/matter in order to be maintained in existence by the organizing principle. Remember that principle 1 states: A universal principle of organization is continually supplying properties and actions to all E/matter, thus maintaining it in existence. Time is continually intrinsic to E/matter through the organizing principle; time will always be "an element necessary" for E/matter to be maintained in existence.

All processes take time (Prin. 6) and the living body does not have infinite time. Vertebral subluxation contributes to further increase the limitation of living E/matter thus further increasing the limits of time already imposed on the body by universal laws including the limitation of time (Prin. 6). This is how the interference occurs with the momentum of the transmission of information/F in the body. The chiropractic objective aims to restore the momentum (timely flow of information/F) of transmission of innate impulses so that the body has maximum time to be re-balanced by the innate law at all levels. The chiropractic objective is about the removal of that interference by locating, analyzing, and facilitating the correction of vertebral subluxations. It is imperative that all human beings, without exception, have their spine checked for vertebral subluxation on a regular basis for their lifetime because eventually we will all run out of time.

ART. 279. THE LAW OF CAUSE AND EFFECT

Vertebral subluxation further increases the limitations of E/matter and time. This is based on another universal law, namely the law of cause and effect. The vertebral subluxation is the cause of a further

71. Bodanis, David. "$E=mc^2$ A Biography of the World's Most Famous Equation." New York, NY: The Berkley Publishing Group. (2000) p. 80-81

72. Densmore, Dana (ed.), "Selections from Newton's Principia" USA:GreenCat Books an imprint of Green Lion Press. (2004) p.23

73. Stephenson, R.W., "Chiropractic Text Book." (Vol XIV) Davenport, IA: The Palmer School of Chiropractic. (1948) p. 239

74. Bodanis, David. "$E=mc^2$ A Biography of the World's Most Famous Equation." New York, NY: The Berkley Publishing Group. (2000) p. 206

increase in limitations of E/matter, which is the effect. To practice the chiropractic objective is to facilitate the correction of that cause, which in turn removes the effect.

The law of cause and effect is very simple. Every effect has a cause and every cause has effects (Prin. 17). Understanding the relationship between cause and effect requires us to philosophically examine the cause, the source of the universal principle of organization. The starting point of chiropractic's basic science is principle 1, namely, "a universal principle of organization is continually supplying properties and actions to all E/matter, thus maintaining it in existence." The verb "is", actually denotes an intrinsic presence of the organizing principle continually supplying properties and actions. It is an act.[75] Furthermore, it is a continual act that maintains E/matter in existence. The act in principle 1 is the universal principle of organization. It is the cause of the effect of E/matter being maintained in existence (Prin. 1), thus manifesting motion ($F = ma$) (Prin. 14). An act logically requires an actor that would be the cause of a cause. The cause of organization is the universal principle of organization. It is the starting point of chiropractic's basic science and comprises the "WHAT" of chiropractic. This begs the question, "What is the cause of the universal principle of organization?" To answer this question, we must rely on chiropractic philosophy, which is the "WHY" of chiropractic.

Chiropractic consists of three aspects, namely, philosophy, science, and art. The universal principle of organization is an act organizing information/F into instructions that supply properties and actions to E/matter in order to maintain E/matter in existence (Prin. 1). It is the core assumption and the starting point of chiropractic's basic science where everything else derives its universal values. It is the a priori statement of chiropractic that is assumed to be true from empirical observation. It is a proven fact of laboratory experiments. It is the first principle of chiropractic's basic science. It is the central reference point from which 32 subsequent principles of chiropractic's basic science are derived. Using chiropractic philosophy, with rational logic, we assert that organization bespeaks intelligence, that there cannot be organization without intelligence. Intelligence is intrinsic to organization. It is absolute philosophy.

"The intelligence function comprises the gathering, evaluation and dissemination of information".[76] Therefore universal organization bespeaks universal intelligence. The universal principle of organization is non-discrete and so is the universal intelligence intrinsic to it non-discrete as well. Philosophically, a universal intelligence is the cause of the universal principle of organization that is the cause of the organization of the universe. It is this organizing principle that is maintaining E/matter in existence (Prin. 1). This begs another question, "What is the cause of a universal intelligence that is the cause of the organizing principle?" Chiropractic does not address this question. It is beyond the realm of chiropractic philosophy, science, and art. "Why, you may ask." Because the starting point of chiropractic's basic science is the universal principle of organization and the science aspect of chiropractic is the "WHAT" of chiropractic. [77]

Chiropractic acknowledges the relationship between cause and effect and between effect and cause. The three aspects of chiropractic, namely, philosophy, science, and art, are separate and distinct from each other, yet the integration of these three aspects are absolutely vital to the existence of chiropractic. Chiropractic cannot exist without its science (basic and applied), without its philosophy, and without its art. The 33 principles of chiropractic's basic science need chiropractic's applied science. The 33 principles must be applied in order to practice the chiropractic objective through the art of chiropractic.

---

75. Stephenson, R.W., "Chiropractic Text Book." (Vol XIV) Davenport, IA: The Palmer School of Chiropractic. (1948) p. 255

76. McDougal, Lassewell, and Reisman. "The Intelligence Function and World Public Order." Temple University of the Commonwealth System of Higher Education. Spring 1973, Vol 46, No 3, p.365

77. Stephenson, R.W., "Chiropractic Text Book." (Vol XIV) Davenport, IA: The Palmer School of Chiropractic. (1948) p. xiv

Chiropractic science (basic and applied) cannot live without chiropractic philosophy otherwise it would lead to mindless activism. Chiropractic's basic science and chiropractic philosophy intersect at the application of innate principles in practice; this means that the principles of chiropractic's basic science and chiropractic philosophy, in practice, have mutual synergy. Chiropractic philosophy needs chiropractic science otherwise chiropractic would remain an empty idealism. Chiropractic cannot exist without the application of its basic science principles, which is the art form of the practice of chiropractic.

No single aspect of chiropractic should be overemphasized , whether its philosophy, its science, or its art. There is a definite need to integrate the three aspects of chiropractic and to study their "relations between Cause and Effect, and Effect and Cause".[78] This relationship between cause and effect may be expressed in the formula: if A is the cause of B and B is the cause of C, then A may also be regarded as the cause of C. In fact, the cause survives in its effect.

An important characteristic of the relationship between cause and effect is its continuous unbroken relational connection. Its chain has neither beginning nor end (Prin. 1). It is never broken. It extends continually from one link to another. Its internal mechanism is associated with the instructive information/F expressed by E/matter and manifested as motion (Prin. 13, 14). It operates everywhere there is existence (Prin. 1), therefore it is universal.

In the context of cause and effect, a universal principle of organization continually supplies instructive information/F to all E/matter causing the unification of the three necessary uniting factors, namely, the organizing principle, information/F, and E/matter (Prin. 1, 3, 4, 10, 17). This is what is called, a hard to vary explanation of the relationship between cause and effect. Through deductive reasoning it leads to the logical and rational conclusion of the chiropractic objective, namely the restoration of transmission of conducted innate information/F through the correction of vertebral subluxations. The study of the 33 principles of chiropractic's basic science has always been known to be about "the relations between Cause and Effect, and Effect and Cause".[79]

ART. 280. EXAMPLES OF USING THE UNIVERSAL LAW OF CAUSE AND EFFECT

All of our actions (cause) have consequences (effect), meaning that we are responsible for our actions as we are responsible for their consequences. Oftentimes we will find excuses so as to not face up with the consequences of our actions. We'll say, "I did not mean it" or "that's not what I really did." However, the law of cause and effect is perfect and immutable. Therefore, no matter how many excuses we bring into a moment, the truth remains the truth. The law of cause and effect is unchangeable, it is what it is. It is a set universal laws caused by the universal principle of organization (Prin. 1, 17).

The question is, "Are you intentionally going to set causes in motion to take charge of your one and only precious life? Or are you going let other people run your life by setting these causes for you? It is you WHO chooses to act or let others act for you. Make no mistake, the law of cause and effect is continuously at work (Prin. 17). It is important to have an understanding of this universal law.

---

78. Stephenson, R.W., "Chiropractic Text Book." (Vol XIV) Davenport, IA: The Palmer School of Chiropractic. (1948) p. 256

79. Stephenson, R.W., "Chiropractic Text Book." (Vol XIV) Davenport, IA: The Palmer School of Chiropractic. (1948) p. 256

We cannot refute the fact that we are responsible for putting the universal law of cause and effect at work for us. It is the same as putting the law of aerodynamics at work for us to fly from New York to Chicago. Cause and effect.

The significance of the law of cause and effect is quite unmistakable. If we attempt to modify what is immutable, we will violate universal laws and we will have to deal with the consequences. Cause and effect. For example, as an accomplished pilot, I can choose to jump out of the plane without a parachute and die as a result of the universal law of gravitation. Or I can use a parachute, using the laws of aerodynamics and descend toward the ground in a safe manner. Cause and effect.

ART. 281. CAUSE AND EFFECT APPLIED TO CRAVINGS AND ADDICTION

Signals of physical cravings and addiction appear contrary to wholeness. Why would a body crave a harmful substance like crack-cocaine or heroin? Is it due to the innate law failing to adapt and compute information/F or E/matter in that circumstance? Of course not, because we have seen that the innate law is 100%/perfect and its function always normal (Prin. 22, 27). The innate law is also always constructive as regard to structural E/matter (Prin. 26).

According to the chiropractic lexicon, a poison is any substance introduced into or manufactured within the living body which the innate law of living things cannot process for metabolism. Suppose you introduce a poison into your body. There will be an immediate computation from the innate law to process this harmful substance in a constructive way by perhaps producing an antidote to neutralize the poison. Cause and effect. The molecular composition of the poison interacts with the molecular composition of the antidote and this action neutralizes the offensive substance. What is fascinating is that the antidote is also a harmful substance, which means that when the poison is no longer present, the antidote may still be in the body. This explains addictions and how the body may crave the toxins to neutralize the antidote that was produced to counteract the harmful substance in the first place. It takes time to evacuate both the poison and the antidote (Prin. 6). Addiction is simply a relationship of molecular compositions warranting continuous interactive computations. Cause and effect. It is a classic example of the innate law adapting information/F and E/matter for the body only if it is possible according to universal laws (Prin. 24). The innate law is limited by the limitations of E/matter and time.

REVIEW QUESTIONS FOR ARTICLES 276 – 281

1. In chiropractic, what is the definition of a principle?
2. What is the cause of all universal laws?
3. Give an example that can predict the behavior of E/matter under certain circumstances.
4. Why is the capability of the innate law to adapt information/F and E/matter limited by time?
5. Why is time an element necessary to the bond between the organizing principle and E/matter?
6. What is the cause of a further increase in limitations of E/matter that chiropractic is addressing?
7. What is the starting point of chiropractic's basic science?
8. Philosophically, what is the cause of the universal principle of organization?
9. How does a chiropractor practice the art form of chiropractic?
10. Give an example of the law of cause and effect at work.
11. Explain addictions from cause and effect.

ART. 282. SYMPTOMS

The universal law of cause and effect, it is time to address and understand an effect of a cause, surprisingly, symptoms. Philosophically, symptoms are a type of information/F from the innate law that may act as feedback for the educated intelligence, signaling that the limitations of E/matter have been reached. Most people use symptoms as an emergency warning system. However, symptoms have their own limitations. The innate law is 100%/perfect and normal (Prin. 22, 27) and uses E/matter that is limited (Prin. 24). If there is a breakdown of E/matter, the limits of adaptation have been passed and symptoms may or may not result. Yet, these symptoms are the effects of a cause which is an increase of the limits of adaptation. What caused the reaching of those limits? From chiropractic's basic science, vertebral subluxation further increases the limitation of E/matter causing incoordination of activities (Prin. 29, 30, 31a). That is why objective chiropractors assert the importance of regular chiropractic care regardless of whether or not symptoms are present.

Symptoms are functional activities of comprised innate information/F and E/matter, computed and coded by the innate law. As such, symptoms are beneficials for use in the body (Prin. 23). They are not the cause of functional activities. They are effects of a cause. They are manifestations of specific computations, by the innate law, in order to adapt the body to keep everything balanced according to universal laws. Chiropractic deal with cause, not effect. Objective chiropractors assert the importance of regular chiropractic care regardless of whether or not symptoms are present.

ART. 283. FUNCTIONALITY OF SYMPTOMS IS NOT A CHIROPRACTIC ISSUE

Chiropractic does not concern itself with effects such as symptoms, which are evidence of physiological change. However, in order to appreciate the irrelevance of symptoms in chiropractic, let us see the reasons for this.

They are two types of symptoms, either an increase in function or a decrease in function. This can be normal or abnormal. In both instances, the 100%/perfect innate law will adapt and compute this information/F in order to adapt the parts of the body that are involved. Symptoms can be objective and subjective. Symptoms can be clinical and subclinical.

Certain functional symptoms produce physiological changes that are experienced as physical signs. For example, the menstrual cycle with its average of 28 days will produce some signs of its functionality. There will be hormonal changes, emotional flux, increase appetite, changes in blood flow, skin complexion changes, and a many other symptoms, known and unknown.

A myriad of cycles goes on simultaneously within the body, moment to moment, causing an assemblage of potentialities and probabilities that defy the imagination. Some effects of these cycles can be symptoms that are uneasy even though they might be exactly as they should be. The educated intelligence cannot determine what is normal. It can only know for sure, from chiropractic's basic science, that only the innate law is always normal and its function is always normal (Prin. 27). Therefore, let us realize that symptoms are not good criteria of assessments, not even to determine the presence or absence of vertebral subluxations.

Symptoms can be objective or subjective. Objective symptoms are observed through an examination of the body by providing a series of tests to determine what is remarkable or not. Subjective symptoms are felt by a person through the five senses and described to another, such as pain for example, whether it be burning pain, stabbing pain, and so forth.

Symptoms can be clinical or subclinical. Clinical symptoms are determined objectively by the examiner or subjectively by the person being examined. Subclinical symptoms are really not symptoms, in so far that they cannot be detected. For example, a lack of absorption of vitamin C may be subclinical for years before it progressed to clinical symptoms that are observable.

Highlighting the magnitude of the complexity of symptomatology reveals the need to discuss this subject. Here are just a few reasons why chiropractic does not concern itself with symptoms.

First, the absence or presence of symptoms may have nothing to do with the absence or presence of vertebral subluxations. Second, symptoms are oftentimes appropriate physiology (menstruation). They are signs of adaptation. Third, people without vertebral subluxations can develop symptoms.

Therefore, with its multitude of simultaneous cycles going on, moment to moment, in the body, it is impossible for the educated intelligence to determine what is normal or what is abnormal with certainty. Only the innate law and its function is normal (Prin. 27). Chiropractic is always about what is possible according to universal laws (Prin. 24).

ART. 284. FALLABILITY OF SYMPTOMS

Symptoms are absolutely useless criteria to determine the presence or absence of vertebral subluxations. The meaning of symptoms depends completely on the limited ability of interpretation of the examiner. Thus, since every examiner is limited, so is the interpretation of symptoms limited. That's where the fall-ability comes from. The assumption that the presence of symptoms is negative and that the absence of symptoms is positive creates a false premise that is refuted by chiropractic. Chiropractic does not concern itself with symptoms. Chiropractic's basic science consists of 33 principles, none of which mentioned symptoms. Chiropractic is separate and distinct from everything else and it is inclusive of everyone regardless of the presence or absence of symptoms.

ART. 285. THE UNKNOWN MEANING OF SYMPTOMS

A symptom may have a certain meaning for someone and another meaning for someone else. A symptom can mean something one day and something else another day in the same person. The physiological changes occurring within the body, moment to moment, reveals that the body is in constant flux of adaptability. Environmental circumstances meet internal processes that are computed under innate control to adapt the living body moment to moment. The physiology of the living body is continuously changing and adapting (Prin. 23, 33) all the time (Prin. 6) and always according to universal laws (Prin. 24). Upon closer observation, symptoms are merely signs that the body is adapting to change.

For example, temperature of a living body is that which is required to meet a particular moment. No one can be certain of what it should be. It is what it is moment to moment. Under certain circumstances the temperature may be more or may be less than the previous moment. Heat is known to be a catalyst that will precipitate chemical reactions. If the body is meeting foreign viruses producing toxins, its internal temperature may rise as a direct result of the innate law computing and adapting the body at this specific moment. In this case, higher temperature is an adaptive body function that is a catalyst to neutralize the toxins in order to protect the body (Prin. 25).

ART. 286. CHIROPRACTIC IS NOT CONCERNED WITH PREVENTION

The same way that chiropractic is not concerned with symptoms, neither is chiropractic concerned with the prevention of symptoms or any other type of prevention. The sole concern of chiropractic is the restoration of the momentum of innate impulse through the correction of vertebral subluxations. The practice of the chiropractic objective allows the living body to function free of vertebral subluxation (Prin. 31a, 31b) in order to fulfill the principle of coordination (Prin. 32). Chiropractic's unique criterion is whether or not the living body is free from vertebral subluxations thereby decreasing the limits of adaptation of E/matter that were further increased by vertebral subluxations. This allows the body to be once again more adaptable and to bring about change. The chiropractic objective is based on the 33 principles of chiropractic's basic science, which reveal the undeniable truth that at all times, a person under all circumstances will have a different experience without nerve interference caused by vertebral subluxation.

ART. 287. CHIROPRACTIC'S CERTAINTY

Chiropractic's basic science asserts that the innate law is 100%/perfect, complete, and normal (Prin. 5, 22, 27). The innate law will adapt, compute, code, and assemble information/F and E/matter for use in the body (Prin. 23). The purpose of the innate law is to maintain the living body alive (Prin. 21). It will never injure or deconstruct the structures in which it works (Prin. 25). It will do so as long as it is possible according to universal laws (Prin. 24, 28, 29, 30, 31a, 31b). Chiropractors aim to restore with certainty the momentum of the transmission of innate impulses by practicing the chiropractic objective (location, analysis, and facilitation of the correction of vertebral subluxations for an innate-normal transmission of innate impulses). Chiropractic is always about what is possible. Chiropractic is always positive for the living body.

ART. 288. INTRODUCTION TO CHIROPRACTIC ANALYSIS

Chiropractic analysis is a process of surveying the spine and its correcting paravertebral muscles to educatedly interpret, to the best of our ability, what the innate law is computing through adaptation to correct a vertebral subluxation. It is our attempt at identifying the cause of nerve interference with the transmission of innate impulses and classifying its working muscles accordingly. It is important to note that it is only the 100%/perfect innate law that controls the normal relationship of the vertebra (Prin. 22, 27). It is only the innate control that can produce a vertebral adjustment according to universal laws (Prin. 23, 24). It is not possible for the educated mind to know where the vertebra belongs in relationship with one another. The unique individual design of each vertebra is too complex and multifaceted for anyone to know. However, since the innate law and its function is always normal (Prin. 27), there is an innate-normal for every innate computation, including the exact position of vertebra in relationship with each other.

Method: The art of using muscle palpation based on the principles of chiropractic's basic science.

The art of muscle palpation evolved from the century old bone palpation developed by D.D. Palmer, the founder of chiropractic, in the late 1890s. It was a crude observation and feeling of bumps along the spine. Eventually bone palpation was used to determine the structures of the vertebra and compare them with a group of five vertebra at a time, according to B.J. Palmer, the developer of chiropractic.[80]

80. Palmer, B.J., "A Text Book on the Palmer Technique of Chiropractic." (Vol XIII) Davenport, IA (1920) p. 34

Bone palpation was done with the subject in a seated position to determine structural information and that necessitated that the person be in an upright position. It is important to note that we have not just refined D.D.'s and B.J.'s palpation, we have developed an analysis that has a totally different purpose. The purpose of muscle palpation is to determine the dynamics of the spinal muscles in relation to the spinal vertebra and the subject is in a relaxed prone position for the analysis. This is to allow the chiropractor to obtain information that is more accurate for the purpose of ascertaining the working muscles involved in the correction of the vertebral subluxation. Volume Four will be an in-depth study of the ADIO analysis that was academically developed in the mid 1970s by Reggie Gold, D.C., and two chiropractic students, Miguel Bolufer and me.

ART. 289. THE PHILOSOPHY OF VERTEBRAL SUBLUXATION

Vertebral subluxation is a philosophical concept because it involves a metaphysical component, which is the interference in transmission of innate impulse from brain cell to tissue cell. From chiropractic's basic science, studies have shown that "A pressure of only 10mm Hg produced a significant conduction block, the potential falling to 60% of its initial value in 15 minutes and to half its initial value in 30 minutes."[81] When the interference with transmission of the conducting nerve cell occurs, the nerve lacks ease (DIS-EASE) and becomes imbalanced due to its impingement. Then the tone of the nerve cell becomes too tense or too slack and cannot properly convey the innate impulse with innate-normal momentum, thus a pivotal moment happens at the site of the impingement. This altered momentum reverts the adapted innate information/F (innate impulse) that is constructive toward structural E/matter to an un-adapted universal information/F (nerve impulse) that is deconstructive toward structural E/matter (Prin. 26). The lack of ease (tone) corrupts the data of the nerve cell through the altered momentum of transmission (Prin. 6). Stephenson wrote it this way, "A nerve cell which is impinged is not a cell 'at ease.' Therefore, it will not 'vibrate' normally in function. Its function is to convey the message. If it does not function properly, it does not carry the 'urge' (momentum) properly, therefore the tissue receives a message, which does not 'read true'."[82] The timing of the transmission the innate impulse though the nerve system for coordination of activities of all the parts of the body is paramount (Prin. 6). There is no exception. That is exactly what chiropractic ensures through the practice of its objective. Nothing more, nothing less, nothing else.

Note to the student: The parts (organs, glands, vessels, etc.) of the body are not dumb or smart. They are biophysical agents expressing the information/F that they receive.

---

81. Sharpless, S.K., "Susceptibility of Spinal Nerve Roots to Compression Block." DHEW Publication (NIH) 767-998, (1975)

82. Stephenson, R.W., "Chiropractic Text Book." (Vol XIV) Davenport, IA: The Palmer School of Chiropractic. (1948) p. 299-300

ART. 290. THE CHIROPRACTIC OBJECTIVE

If an initial principle is true and we use rational logic with sound deductive reasoning, its subsequent principles and conclusion will also be true. "Chiropractic is a deductive science";[83] therefore, the 33 principles of chiropractic's basic science should reveal the chiropractic objective. The scientific application of the 33 principles, in practice, is actually chiropractic's applied science, through the art of chiropractic in practice, with its analyses/techniques including the educational programs for practice members. Chiropractic is a complete science.[84] Therefore, let us apply some of the principles to see clearly the chiropractic objective:

No. 13. The function of Energy/Matter

The function of E/matter is to express information/F.

No. 20. Innate Law of Living Things

A living thing has an inborn organizing principle governing its body, called the innate law of living things.

No. 21. The Purpose of the Innate Law of Living Things

The purpose of the innate law of living things is to maintain the material of the body of a living thing alive.

No. 22. The Quality of the Innate Law of Living Things

The innate law of living things is always 100%/perfect for all living energy/matter.

No. 23. The Function of the Innate Law of Living Things

The function of the innate law of living things is to adapt universal information/force and energy/matter for use in the body, so that all parts of the body will have coordinated action for mutual benefit.

No. 24. The limits of Adaptation

The innate law of living things adapts information/force for the body only if it is possible according to universal laws.

No. 25. The Character of Innate Information/Force

The information/force of the innate law of living things never injures or deconstructs the structures in which it works.

---

83. Stephenson, R.W., "Chiropractic Text Book." (Vol XIV) Davenport, IA: The Palmer School of Chiropractic. (1948) p. 299-300

84. Stephenson, R.W., "Chiropractic Text Book." (Vol XIV) Davenport, IA: The Palmer School of Chiropractic. (1948) p. xvi

No. 26. Comparison of Universal Information/Force and Innate Information/Force

In order to carry on the universal cycle of life, universal information/force is deconstructive, and innate information/force is reconstructive, regarding structural energy/matter.

No. 27. The Normality of the Innate Law of Living Things

The innate law of living things is always normal and its function is always normal.

No. 28. The Conductors of Innate Information/Force

The conducted information/force of the innate law of living things operates through or over the nervous system in animal bodies.

No. 29. Interference with Transmission of Conducted Innate Information/Force

There can be interference with the transmission of conducted innate information/force.

No. 30. The Cause of DIS-EASE

Interference with transmission of conducted innate information/force causes incoordination of DIS-EASE.

No. 31. The Vertebral Subluxation and its Correction

a. The vertebral subluxation is the uniquely chiropractic entity as a cause of interference to the transmission of conducted innate information/force,

b. and the correction of a vertebral subluxation is always due to the process of adapting information/force by the innate law of living things.

No. 32. The Principle of Coordination

Coordination is the principle of coherent actions of all the parts of an organism in fulfilling their roles and purposes.

No. 33. The principle of Continuous Supply and Computation

The principle of continuous supply and computation is existent in the body in its ideal state wherein the living body is the "computer," the innate law is the "normal software," the innate field is the "operating system," the brain is the "central processing unit," the brain cells are the "processors", and the nerve cells are the "transmitters."

Using deductive reasoning and rational logic, we observe that the conclusion of the principles of chiropractic's basic science does reveal the exclusive chiropractic objective. Stated: The chiropractic objective is to locate, analyze and facilitate the correction of vertebral subluxations (Prin. 30, 31a, 31b) for an innate-normal (Prin. 27) transmission of the conducted innate information/F of the body (Prin. 29). An initial draft of the chiropractic objective first appeared within the objective straight chiropractic lexicon found in the blog called "Chiropractic Outside the Box" (COTB), April 22, 2014.[85] In those days, we were just beginning to "see" something new, to "see" something we never "saw" before. We realized then, that the chiropractic objective stemmed from the view point of E/matter expressing innate information/F. Stephenson somewhat identified the chiropractic objective when he wrote, "The chiropractor aims only to restore – to bring about restoration."[86]

ART. 291. THE CHIROPRATIC OBJECTIVE AND E/MATTER

The function of E/matter is to express information/F that is governed by the universal principle of organization (Prin. 13). Information/F is instruction supplying properties (configurations) and actions (velocities) to the electrons, protons, and neutrons in the interest of maintaining E/matter in existence (Prin. 1) uniting the organizing principle with E/matter (Prin. 3, 10). Progressing to more complex levels of organization, recognize that an essential extension of the universal principle of organization, which is the innate law of living things, is adapting universal information/F and E/matter to maintain the material of the body of a living thing alive (Prin. 21) within the limitations of E/matter (Prin. 24) and of time (Prin. 6). The innate law is always 100%/perfect and complete (Prin. 22). The innate law governs living E/matter and is either 100% active or it is 0%. If it has 0% of activity it means that E/matter is dead. There is no in-between with the innate law. It is all (100%) or it is nothing (0%). A thing is alive or it is dead. It is never possible for living E/matter to express more of the innate law. It cannot be said that the chiropractic objective is to express more innate. It is the innate law that is the governing principle[87] and it is always 100% (Prin. 22). The correction of vertebral subluxation, which is the fundamental of the chiropractic objective, allows the living E/matter of the body to express innate-normal information /F for use in the body and coordination of activities if it is possible according to universal laws (Prin. 13, 23, 24, 27, 29, 31a, 31b).

ART. 292. THE CHIROPRACTIC OBJECTIVE AND THE LAW OF CAUSE AND EFFECT

The nerve system conducts innate information/F (innate impulses) for coordination of activities of all the parts of the body (Prin. 28). There can be interference with the transmission of conducted innate information/F (Prin. 29). Interference with transmission of conducted innate information/F causes incoordination of DIS-EASE (Prin. 30). The vertebral subluxation is the uniquely chiropractic entity as a cause of interference to the transmission of conducted innate information/F (Prin. 31a). The correction of a vertebral subluxation is always due to the process of the adapting information/F by the innate control to process a vertebral adjustment (Prin. 31b). However, since the function of E/matter is to express information/F, the expression of information/F by E/matter is an effect and not a cause.

85. Strauss, Joseph. Chiropractic Outside of the Box Blog- Objective Straight Chiropractic Lexicon. April 22, 2014. josephbstrauss.com/updated-lexicon (03/2022)

86. Stephenson, R.W., "Chiropractic Text Book." (Vol XIV) Davenport, IA: The Palmer School of Chiropractic. (1948) p. 270

87. Stephenson, R.W., "Chiropractic Text Book." (Vol XIV) Davenport, IA: The Palmer School of Chiropractic. (1948) p. 18

Stephenson wrote, "Chiropractic is a science of cause --- not effects."[88] Through rational logic and sound deductive reasoning, for the chiropractic objective to be congruent, it must be based on the principles of its basic "science of cause." Art. 290 illustrated the chiropractic objective must be about bringing restoration[89] namely, the restoration of transmission of conducted information/F back to innate-normal through the correction of vertebral subluxations (Prin. 27, 28, 29, 31a, 31b).

When you, as a chiropractor, have located, analyzed, and facilitated the correction of vertebral subluxations, you have participated in the correction of the cause of DIS-EASE (Prin. 30, 31a, 31b). You have fulfilled the purpose of chiropractic and your work is thus completed. You have practiced the chiropractic objective. You are an objective chiropractor.

88. Stephenson, R.W., "Chiropractic Text Book." (Vol XIV) Davenport, IA: The Palmer School of Chiropractic. (1948) p. 93

89. Stephenson, R.W., "Chiropractic Text Book." (Vol XIV) Davenport, IA: The Palmer School of Chiropractic. (1948) p. 270

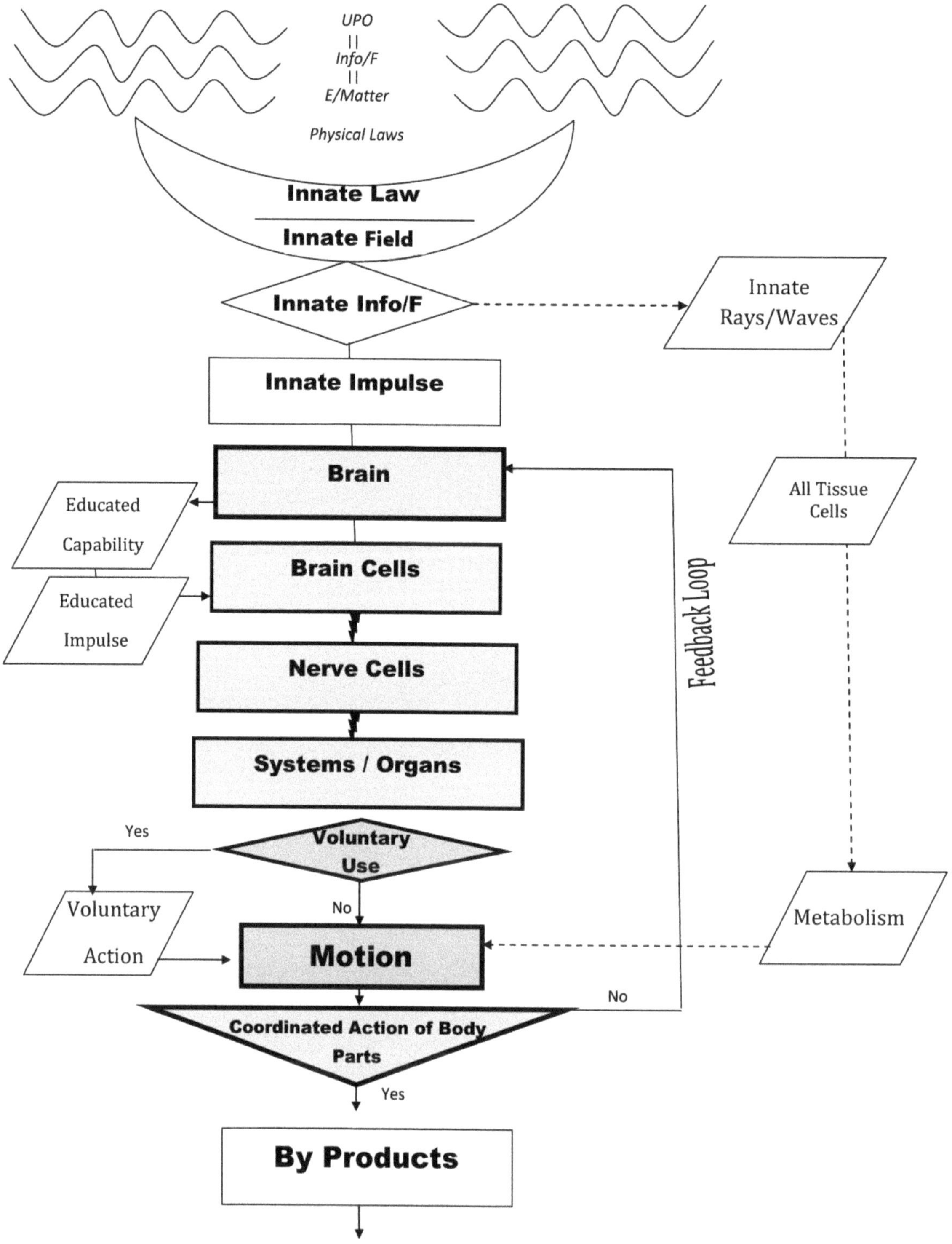

Fig 35: Flowchart of the innate law of living vertebrates adapting information/F and E/matter for use in the body through innate control of cellular components for metabolism radiating innate rays/waves within all tissue cells; for coordination of actions of all body parts through innate control conducting transmission of innate impulses through the nervous system; for voluntary actions through educated control conducting transmission of tinctured innate impulses into educated impulses through the nervous system. It also depicts the interference with transmission of conducted innate information/F located within the transmitting nerve cells. The feedback loop is the necessary communication system exclusively for the control of coordinated action of all parts of the body for mutual benefit (Prin. 23).

This is the conclusion of Volume Three (third year junior text).

Proceed to Volume Four

BIBLIOGRAPHY VOL 3:

1. Strauss, Joseph. "The Green Book Commentaries, Vol. XIV (1927) Chiropractic Text Book." Levittown, PA: Foundation for Advancement of Chiropractic Education. (2002). p.17

2. Palmer, B.J., " The Science of Chiropractic, Its Principles and Philosophies." 4th ed., Davenport, IA: The Palmer School of Chiropractic- Chiropractic Fountain Head. (1920) p. 12

25. Palmer, D.D., "Text-Book of the Science, Art, and Philosophy of Chiropractic for Students and Practioners." Portland, OR: Portland Printing House Company. (1910) p. 7

36. https://www.nids.nih.gov/health-information/public-education/brain-basics-life-and-death-neuron#:~:text=A%20%20has%20three%20three%20basic,sends%20messages%20from%20the%20cell (Feb 25, 2025).

37. Sundermier, Ali. "The Particle Physics of You." symmetrymagazine.org/articlethe-particle-physics-of-you?language_content_entity=und (Nov 3, 2025).

38. Palmer, B.J., "The Bigness of the Fellow Within" (Vol 22) Davenport, IA: Chiropractic Fountainhead (1949) p. 21

39. López-Muñoz, F, Alamo, C, "Historical Evolution of the Neurotransmission Concept." Journal of Neural Transmission, 2009 May; 116:515-33

40. Stephenson, R.W., "Chiropractic Text Book." (Vol XIV) Davenport, IA: The Palmer School of Chiropractic. (1948) p. 9,11

41. Stephenson, R.W., "Chiropractic Text Book." (Vol XIV) Davenport, IA: The Palmer School of Chiropractic. (1948) p. 13-15

42. Wong, L, Cleland,C.E., et al. "On the Roles of Function and Selection in Evolviing Systems." PNAS Vol. 120, No. 43 (2023) doi: 10.1073.2310223120

43. Palmer, D.D., editior B.J. Palmer. "The Chiropractic Adjuster." Davenport, IA: The Palmer School of Chiropractic. (1921) p. 772

44. Funk, Richard H.W., "Understanding the Feedback Loops Between Energy, Matter, and Life." Front.Biosci. (Elite Ed.) 2022, 14(4)29. doi: 10.310083/j.fbe1404029

45. Palmer, B.J., "Chiropractic Clinical Controlled Research." Davenport, IA: Chiropractic Fountain Head. (1951) p. 219-220

46. Tamura, Koji. "The Genetic Code: Francis Crick's Legacy and Beyond" Life 2016; 6(3):36 doi: 10.3390/life6030036

47. Sharpless, S.K., "Susceptibility of Spinal Nerve Roots to Compression Block." DHEW Publication (NIH) 767-998, (1975)

48. Sharpless, S.K., "Susceptibility of Spinal Nerve Roots to Compression Block." DHEW Publication (NIH) 767-998, (1975)

49. Hynes, R.J.R., Callender A.K. "Technique in the Classroom at Palmer College of Chiropractic: A history of art in chiropractic." J Chirophuman 2008; 15:55-66

50. "The Triune of Life: Reggie Gold's Philosophical Legacy." Senzon, Simon (ed.) Asheville, NC: The Institute Chiropractic. (2022) p.xix-xx

51. Densmore, Dana (ed.), "Selections from Newton's Principia" USA:GreenCat Books an imprint of Green Lion Press. (2004) p.31

52. Ashtekar, Berger, Isenberg, and MacCallum (eds.) "Gravity is Geometry, after all. General Relativity and Gravation: A Centennial Perspective." Cambridge: Cambridge University Press. (2015) p. 347 doi: 10.1017/CB09781139583961.010

53. Stephenson, R.W., "Chiropractic Text Book." (Vol XIV) Davenport, IA: The Palmer School of Chiropractic. (1948) p. 13

54. Field Programmable Gate Array (FPGA) xilinx.com/products/silicon-devices/fpga/what-is-an-fpga.html (Jan 2021)

55. The Synpase. Khanacademy.org/science/biology/human-biology/neuron-nervous-system/a/the-synapse (2021)

56. Lessard, Claude. "A New Look at Chiropractic's Basic Science." (2014) Self Published. p.59

57. Palmer, B.J., "The Value of Chiropractic." (1915) Davenport, IA: The Palmer School of Chiropractic Fountain Head. (1997 Reprint) p. 19-20

58. Palmer, D.D., "The Chiropractic Adjuster. The Science, Art, and Philosophy of Chiropractic." Portland, OR: Portland Printing House. (1910) p. 1

59. Palmer, D.D., "The Chiropractic Adjuster. The Science, Art, and Philosophy of Chiropractic." Portland, OR: Portland Printing House. (1910) p. 280

60. Field Programmable Gate Array (FPGA) xilinx.com/products/silicon-devices/fpga/what-is-an-fpga.html (Jan 2021)

61. Synapse. The Encyclopaedia Britannica. Britannica.com/science/synapse (Jan 27, 2025)

62. Zyga, Lisa. "Quantum No-hiding Theorem Experimentally Confirmed for First Time." Phys.org News (03/07/2011). https://phys.org/news/2011-03-quantum-no-hiding-theorem-experimentally.html (viewed 03/03/2025)

63. Jharana, Rani, Samal, et al. "Experimental Test of Quantum No-hiding Theorem." Phys Review Letters. 106, 080401 (2011) doi: 10.1103/PhysRevLett.106.080401

64. Zyga, Lisa. "Quantum No-hiding Theorem Experimentally Confirmed for First Time." Phys.org News (03/07/2011). https://phys.org/news/2011-03-quantum-no-hiding-theorem-experimentally.html (viewed 03/03/2025)

65. DNA Replication. www.genome.gov/genetics-glossary/DNA-replication (03/03/2025)

66. Sharpless, S.K., "Susceptibility of Spinal Nerve Roots to Compression Block." DHEW Publication (NIH) 767-998, (1975)

67. Palmer, D.D., "Text-Book of the Science, Art, and Philosophy of Chiropractic for Students and Practioners." Portland, OR: Portland Printing House Company. (1910) p. 7

68. Densmore, Dana (ed.), "Selections from Newton's Principia" USA:GreenCat Books an imprint of Green Lion Press. (2004) p. 31

69. Ashtekar, Berger, Isenberg, and MacCallum (eds.) "Gravity is Geometry, after all. General Relativity and Gravation: A Centennial Perspective." Cambridge: Cambridge University Press. (2015) p. 347 doi: 10.1017/CB09781139583961.010

70. Stephenson, R.W., "Chiropractic Text Book." (Vol XIV) Davenport, IA: The Palmer School of Chiropractic. (1948) p. 2, 320

71. Bodanis, David. "$E=mc^2$ A Biography of the World's Most Famous Equation." New York, NY: The Berkley Publishing Group. (2000) p. 80-81

72. Densmore, Dana (ed.), "Selections from Newton's Principia" USA:GreenCat Books an imprint of Green Lion Press. (2004) p. 23

73. Stephenson, R.W., "Chiropractic Text Book." (Vol XIV) Davenport, IA: The Palmer School of Chiropractic. (1948) p. 239

74. Bodanis, David. "$E=mc^2$ A Biography of the World's Most Famous Equation." New York, NY: The Berkley Publishing Group. (2000) p. 206

75. Stephenson, R.W., "Chiropractic Text Book." (Vol XIV) Davenport, IA: The Palmer School of Chiropractic. (1948) p. 255

76. McDougal, Lassewell, and Reisman. "The Intelligence Function and World Public Order." Temple University of the Commonwealth System of Higher Education. Spring 1973, Vol 46, No 3, p. 365

77. Stephenson, R.W., "Chiropractic Text Book." (Vol XIV) Davenport, IA: The Palmer School of Chiropractic. (1948) p. xiv

78. Stephenson, R.W., "Chiropractic Text Book." (Vol XIV) Davenport, IA: The Palmer School of Chiropractic. (1948) p. 256

79. Stephenson, R.W., "Chiropractic Text Book." (Vol XIV) Davenport, IA: The Palmer School of Chiropractic. (1948) p. 256

80. Palmer, B.J., "A Text Book on the Palmer Technique of Chiropractic." (Vol XIII) Davenport, IA (1920) p. 34

81. Sharpless, S.K., "Susceptibility of Spinal Nerve Roots to Compression Block." DHEW Publication (NIH) 767-998, (1975)

82. Stephenson, R.W., "Chiropractic Text Book." (Vol XIV) Davenport, IA: The Palmer School of Chiropractic. (1948) p. 299-300

83. Stephenson, R.W., "Chiropractic Text Book." (Vol XIV) Davenport, IA: The Palmer School of Chiropractic. (1948) p. 299-300

84. Stephenson, R.W., "Chiropractic Text Book." (Vol XIV) Davenport, IA: The Palmer School of Chiropractic. (1948) p. xvi

85. Strauss, Joseph. Chiropractic Outside of the Box Blog- Objective Straight Chiropractic Lexicon. April 22, 2014. josephbstrauss.com/updated-lexicon (03/2022)

86. Stephenson, R.W., "Chiropractic Text Book." (Vol XIV) Davenport, IA: The Palmer School of Chiropractic. (1948) p. 270

87. Stephenson, R.W., "Chiropractic Text Book." (Vol XIV) Davenport, IA: The Palmer School of Chiropractic. (1948) p. 18

88. Stephenson, R.W., "Chiropractic Text Book." (Vol XIV) Davenport, IA: The Palmer School of Chiropractic. (1948) p. 93

89. Stephenson, R.W., "Chiropractic Text Book." (Vol XIV) Davenport, IA: The Palmer School of Chiropractic. (1948) p. 270

CURRICULUM VITAE
DR. CLAUDE LESSARD

- B.S. Limestone College, Gaffney, S.C. 1977
- Doctor Of Chiropractic Degree, Sherman College Of Straight Chiropractic (S.C.S.C), Spartanburg, S.C. 1977
- Internship, S.C.S.C. 1977
- Recipient Of The B.J. Palmer Chiropractic Philosophy Distinction Award, S.C.S.C. 1977
- Diplomate Of The National Board Of Chiropractic Examiners
- Certified For Preliminary Professional Education #C35301, Commonwealth Of Pennsylvania
- Commonwealth Of Pennsylvania License #DC-1702-L
- Co-Founder And Charter Member Of ADIO Institute Of Straight Chiropractic 1978
- Student Referral Counselor, ADIO I.S.C. 1978-1981
- Assistant Professor Of Chiropractic Philosophy, ADIO I.S.C. 1978-1980
- Co-Developer of The ADIO Analysis 1978
- Administrative Dean Of ADIO I.S.C. 1979-1980
- Associate Professor Of Chiropractic Technique, ADIO I.S.C. 1980-1981
- Director Community Health Center, ADIO I.S.C. 1980-1981
- Member Chiropractic Life Fellowship Of Pennsylvania
- Member Of The Federation Of Straight Chiropractors Organization (F.S.C.O.)
- Graduate Of Church Ministry Program, St. Charles Borromeo Seminary 1983-1987
- Certified Myotech Examiner
- Chiropractor Of The Month Award, Markson Management Services, 1988
- Chiropractor Of The Year Award, Markson Management Services, 1992
- Post Graduate Course Of Study In Applied Spinal Biomechanics From The Aragona Spinal Biomechanic Engineering Laboratory, Inc. 1992
- Chiropractor Of The Year Award, Quest Management Systems, 1993
- Member Of The Distinguished Board Of Regents, S.C.S.C. Since 1993
- Member Of Parker Chiropractic Resources Foundation
- Chair And Co-Author Of "Spirit Of '76", S.C.S.C. 1996
- Founder Of Clients Association For Chiropractic Education (C.A.C.E.), 1997
- Licensed Private Pilot, Single Engine Airplanes Land, 1998
- Founder Of Lessard Institute For Chiropractic Clients, 1998
- Recipient Of The Spirit Of Sherman College Of Straight Chiropractic Award, 1999
- Licensed Pilot, Instrument Airplanes, 2000
- Author Of "Chiropractic.... Amazing Isn't It?" 2003
- Chiropractor Of The Year, S.C.S.C., 2006
- Motion De Felicitations, Ville De Ste. Anne De Beaupre, Resolutions 5553-09-06., 2006
- Pulstar Examiner, 2008

- Translation Of “Chiropractic…Amazing Isn’t It?” In French, 2008
- Translation Of “Chiropractic…Amazing Isn’t It?” In Spanish, 2009
- Autor Del Libro “Quiropraxia No Es Asombrosa?” 2010
- Auteur Du Livre “La Chiropratique, Incroyable N’est-Ce Pas?” 2012
- Author Of Blue Book “A New Look At Chiropractic Basic Science” 2017
- Autor Del Libro Azul “Una Mirada A La Scienca Basica Quiropractica” 2019
- Keynote Speaker At Sherman College Of Chiropractic International Research And Philosophy Symposium, 2019
- Author Of “Chiropractic, Amazing Isn’t It- Workbook” 2020
- Author of Blue Book “Timed Out: Chiropractic” 2022
- Autor Del Libro Azul “Quiropráctica Reseteada” 2023
- Author Of “The 2027 Chiropractic Textbook Volume 1” 2024
- Autor Del Libro “Libro de Texto de Quiropráctica 2027 Volume 1” 2024
- Author Of “The 2027 Chiropractic Textbook Volume 2” 2025
- Autor Del Libro “Libro de Texto de Quiropráctica 2027 Volume 2” 2025

www.ingramcontent.com/pod-product-compliance
Ingram Content Group UK Ltd.
Pitfield, Milton Keynes, MK11 3LW, UK
UKHW060221061026
15625UKWH00007B/437

9 798990 012974